Your Pain, My Pleasure
Inside the Mind of a Sexual Sadist
by
FifthAngel

Contributing Authors:
Rich Dockter
Travis Wilson
Hook
Sherrye Segura
slave leslie

Illustrations:
Devin Wilson
Sherrye Segura

Photographs:
Barbara Nitke

CAUTION: The activities described in this book carry some risk of physical or emotional injury, as do most activities in BDSM. While the author has made every attempt to communicate awareness of such risks, it is up to you to accept personal responsibility for all activities you decide to practice. In acting on the information in this book, you agree to accept that information as is and with all faults. Neither the author nor any persons associated with the development or distribution of this book are responsible for any injuries or damages. Some activities described were performed by trained professionals, and should not be attempted by unqualified persons.

All records required by 18 U.S.C. Section 2257 are in the custody of Barbara Nitke, 300 East 34 Street, #6B, New York, NY 10016. Date of Production August 31, 2003.

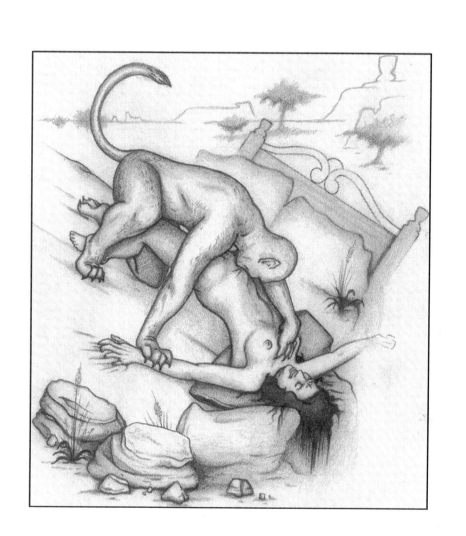

Acknowledgements

This is actually the second printing of the book - the first was in 2006. Shortly after the release of the first printing, my life began to go through significant changes. Most of these changes occurred with the relationships I was in. Rather than bore you every detail of my life, I will give you a brief summary.

My relationships with Leslie and Sherrye ended, two of the contributing authors in the book, and I met my wife Katie. I want to acknowledge Katie first because of the strain a book like this can have on a marriage.

There are some very detailed sexual encounters in this book, stories of past slaves, intense scenes and girlfriends. Some have referred to some sections as "one handed." The intent of the book is to educate you and not to get you off. This was a byproduct that I did not think of. But some of you people are sick fucks.

In my heart I feel it important to educate the BDSM community on what I feel sadism is. I think the subject is best taught by relating my real life stories to you. Katie and I have a "power-balanced" monogamous marriage. These are stories that many monogamous wives would rather not know about. Certainly I can not blame her for this.

It is the past however and it is what has helped shape me into what I am now. I do not regret those relationships, nor do I feel that they should be hidden away. Katie is a very strong woman for working with me and coming to the decision to re-release this book. I love her deeply for this.

I am compelled to thank my contributing authors. If they had not trusted me with their emotional and physical well-being, this book would have never been written. They will provide you with accounts of what it is like to be on the receiving end of sadism.

What kind of sexual sadist would I be without people who let me be mean to them? In the same vein as my contributing authors are the slaves, submissives, and bottoms that I have had the pleasure and honor of working with. Over the years, I have met some truly beautiful people who gave me every ounce of their being. My only regret is that I could not write about all of them here.

Once again Gary Switch and Bob Miller were my editors. They kept telling me that I write well, as I continued to struggle to explain what sadism is to me. I am sure this book was more difficult for them, given the concepts and ideas. It is with their help and that of Leslie that we were able to express what is inside me. It can be tough for a person like me to be submissive to three editors at the same time. Often I found myself giving in while stating "whatever" as I breathed heavily and slumped back in my chair – at least that's how it was with Bob and Gary. With Leslie, she'd make a suggestion, I'd give her at least three reasons why she was wrong while having a ten-minute fit, and then go ahead and make her changes anyway – remember, I'm a sadist.

For this book I thought "why break up a great team?" This time I chose to showcase my friend and self-proclaimed "official photographer" Barbara Nitke on the cover. Devin Wilson, an adopted brother so to speak, provided most of the illustrations. Sherrye Segura provided the illustration for her written contribution. Some of the illustrations were based on photos that Barbara had taken of my scenes. These artists provide a wonderful graphic interpretation of sadism and what it is to me, as well as the spirituality contained within it.

Prologue

I tied Sherrye's limbs to the bed with my trademark purple rope. This made her very nervous since I had never before restrained her. With each consecutive sex session I have with Sherrye, the intensity escalates, and it is always something different. She never has any idea what I will be doing.

I began to slowly insert 5/8-inch-long sterile needles into her fingertips. Even though she was restrained, I had to forcefully hold down her hand as she cried out in pain with each subsequent needle. As she moaned in pain, flashes of how to be even more sadistic ran through my mind. I left her thumbs untouched, yet shoved needles into the tips of both of her big toes – something that had entered my mind while hearing her suffer.

I untied her and watched her lie perfectly still as she whimpered in agony. I was sure she was afraid to move since she might bump a needle into something, resulting in even worse pain. But that was what I wanted her to do.

"Let's see how much you want my blood; come over to me," I whispered in her ear.

My cock was already hard as I sat in a chair about five feet away from the foot of the bed. Beside me on a table were syringes with needles attached. I watched anxiously as she carefully sat up in the bed trying ever so hard not to hit any of the needles jutting out from her fingertips. She was in an intense predicament since she could not use her hands and feet in normal fashion. Each movement had to be precise or she would feel more pain. She made it to the edge of the bed and managed to get to her feet relatively unscathed. Then she bumped her foot on the chair next to me. I winced and laughed at the same time, as I curled up my toes in sympathy. Damn, that had to hurt!

She knelt down in front of me, still writhing in pain. This was a slow process in itself since she could not use her toes to help her kneel and could use only her palms for balance as she kept her fingers arched upward to avoid touching anything. She had proven that she had a love for blood and a love for me.

She watched intently as I drew blood from my right arm. Holding my hard cock in my hand, I dripped blood onto the tip and watched it drip down the sides. I could feel the anticipation building in Sherrye since she now knew what her reward would be. I pulled her face towards me and she began to lick and suck every drop of blood from me. When it was gone, she wanted more. Each time I dripped more blood on me, she became more aggressive as I held my own cock. It seemed her only focus in life at that moment was getting as much blood as she could from me.

She was happy, but I was not.

I took her hands and wrapped them forcefully around my cock. Again, she was in pain as she had great difficulty not pushing the needles further into her fingertips as she masturbated me with my own blood. She was getting what she desired: my blood. I was getting what I desired: her suffering. We drifted in and out of pain and pleasure.

Table of Contents

Acknowledgements 4
Prologue...7
Illustrations 10
Introduction 11
A History of Sadism..15
One Sick Puppy 31
What Are You Thinking? 37
The Lighter Side of SM..44
Masters, slaves, and SM Sex 49
A Word About Safewords..60
Facing Fears..70
More Sadistic Techniques 78
The Other Side of Pain...83
The View from the Bottom:
Pain and Catharsis in the Big Scene by Rich Dockter 89
The Big Scene: Unexpected Lessons in Life.....................110
Another Remembered Piercing by Travis Wilson....................124
Kings Really Do Swing by Travis Wilson.............................128
Inexorable, Continuous, Synchronistic by Hook 135
Finding Release Beyond the Pain by Sherrye Segura 144
Living with a Sexual Sadist by slave leslie 162
The Aftermath...186
About the Authors 196
Glossary 202

Illustrations

FifthAngel as "Sparkie the Clown" and his wife Katie - Original Photo by Barbara Nitke..Cover

Bedroom Sahara - by Devin Wilson...3

Ascension - by Devin Wilson... 102

Inside, Out - by Devin Wilson...126

Floating Warrior - by Devin Wilson...132

Hook Transcendent - by Devin Wilson...140

Swept Away - by Sherrye Segura... 156

1763 - by Devin Wilson..180

Introduction

First, let me make the distinction between sadism and just plain cruelty. Pulling the wings off a fly to see it crawl in misery is not sadism. If you like kicking a dog for no other reason than it makes you happy, you are not a sadist. However, if it makes your pussy wet or your cock hard when you are caning the ass of your partner and they are in pain, you might be a sadist.

Second, I would like to emphasize that what I do is done with consenting people. Unlike the victims of sadistic serial rapists preying on unsuspecting women and men, my partners are willing to engage in scenes with me knowing that my intention is to do things to them that they won't like. In this book, I speak to you as a consensual sadist. From here on out, when I say "sadist," it is to imply consensual sadist unless stated otherwise.

Frequently over the years, I have been asked how I became a sadist. Or what I think when I do what I do. Some people have even asked me to help them with their own sadism. This led to my developing a class called "Awakening the Sadist Within," in which I give practical demonstrations and answer questions. It was during my classes that I learned sadism is largely misunderstood – as is BDSM's original meaning, to a lesser degree.

Let me break down the letters in BDSM. Bondage and Discipline do not have to be about sex, but they can be. Dominance and Submission – again, sex is not a requirement, but it is not prohibited (unless the dominant says so). However, Sadism and Masochism are about sex and only sex. When I asked attendees whether sadism was about sex or not, "No" was one of the common answers I got. But the very origins and definition of the term sadism are about sexual gratification.

It is hard to be a sadist without someone to have sex with and do mean things to. Now not all of my scenes entail actual penetration or even orgasms, but they are still sexually arousing to me. So whether I have some type of sex in a scene or later fuck the hell out of my slave in the hotel room after the dungeon closes, it helps to have someone who lets me cause pain.

You will get a chance to read the stories of several partners I have had experiences with. Some of these encounters were about sadism and others were about catharsis and self-exploration. I feel that, because I am a sadist, it allows me to branch out into other areas of inflicting pain. The essays contained in this book are written by a diverse group of individuals. You will hear from a gay male, a "straight" female who happens to enjoy strap-on sex with lesbians, a bisexual female, a heterosexual male, and one "confused" male. It is my intent, with their help, to give you insight into what makes me tick and why people let me do mean things to them.

The Making of a Sadist

My first self-exploration with what could be called BDSM came after watching the movie Enter The Dragon, starring Bruce Lee. I doubt there's a single martial artist who hasn't seen this movie. What got to me most was the scene where Bruce Lee's character is slashed across the chest by a multi-bladed weapon the villain wears strapped to his arm. The wounds' appearance as perfectly symmetrical lines, glistening with Lee's blood, turned me on so much that I had to see what it would look like on myself. It had nothing to do with martial arts or the desire to mutilate or scar my own flesh. Rather, I saw it as artwork made from the human body – the superbly toned body of an athlete, his bronzed skin contrasting with the brilliant red slashes, perfectly aligned.

Watching the steel as it parted my own flesh and witnessing the blood dripping from me was more erotic than I could ever have imagined. The sensations did not turn me on as much as the visualization of marking my body did. Soon after began my fascination with the fluid of life and the potential of using the human body as a canvas for art.

My first glimpse of BDSM was in the mid-eighties at an ostensibly "vanilla" house party of all places. I was wandering through the various rooms when I stumbled into one where there were flogging and knife scenes taking place. My immediate response was to start to shut the door so as to not to disturb anyone. The traditional, "Oops, sorry I didn't know this room was taken!" crossed my mind, but nobody seemed to care. Remaining silent, I scrunched down and sat on the floor at the base of the bed near the wall. What really caught my eye was the knife scene in the corner. Having delved into scarification already on my own using blades, I was quickly absorbed into the scene. The top was not cutting his partner's skin but was instead using the knife's tip to scrape the surface, leaving little red welts. The bottom was trapped in the corner and unrestrained – they appeared to be enjoying the activity. "You mean there are people who let you do this to them and they like it?" I thought in amazement. "Man did I walk into the right room!" As I got to know more people and explored other activities, my interest in what I would someday learn would be called "BDSM" grew.

Origins of an Angel

Often I am asked where my name comes from. Here is the disclaimer: I have no intent to offend any Christians or church-going folks. I am not really an angel from Hell. This is my nickname and nothing more, although some bottoms may disagree. Sound okay?

Back in 1986 when I first began topping within the BDSM lifestyle, I was very much into inflicting intense pain. I speak of very slow, drawn-out pain over hours – such pain that causes one to think of the pleasures of life…or death.

It was during this time that I heard the band Fifth Angel from Seattle, Washington. When I first heard their music, I was very drawn to it. Each song seemed to be about a different aspect of my life at the time.

The idea of the "Fifth Angel" comes from the book of Revelations. Ironically, there are a few passages concerning death and how men shall seek it for relief from pain and suffering. These are the passages for which I was named.

REV 9:1 And the fifth angel sounded, and I saw a star fall from heaven unto the earth: and to him was given the key of the bottomless pit.

By rite of passage, I was given the privilege to cause others pain and pleasure. I was given the key and my name.

REV 9:5 And to them it was given that they should not kill them, but that they should be tormented five months: and their torment was as the torment of a scorpion, when he striketh a man.

This was parallel to my slow drawn out pain of "pressure points" – the touch of my hand equal to the sting of the scorpion, some would say.

REV 9:6 And in those days shall men seek death, and shall not find it; and shall desire to die, and death shall flee from them.

There are scenes where pain can be so intense that one wishes for death but is denied the relief. When the other side of pain is reached, it is beyond words, a release so cathartic it will change one's life.

I hope this essay has not caused others to think ill thoughts of me. It is the explanation for my given name in the Scene. I do use pain as a means of opening the gateway. Pain can be a good thing, unlike what was written in the Bible.

Am I a true sadist as these verses portray? Does my name still hold true to this day? Perhaps those questions are best answered by my partners and my slave.

A History of Sadism

"The ravished girls were led away to marriage; their very shame made them more beautiful. And when one struggled hard against her captor, He carried her away in eager arms, And said: 'Why spoil your pretty eyes by weeping? Your father took your mother, I take you!'"
(Publius Ovidius Naso, 43 B.C.–17 A.D.)

I selected this poem to bring to your attention the second, third, and fourth lines. It would seem to the eyes of the poet that the psychological shame of the girls made them more attractive and maybe even sexually aroused the onlookers. Unmistakably, when the girl struggled knowing she was going to have sex, possibly forced, her captor was still happy. It is safe to say sex has been around a long time, right? Is it inconceivable that sexual gratification from the suffering of others has been around just as long?

The behavior that we know today as sadism has been around for thousands of years. But it seems there wasn't a name for it until recently. Could it be that this was just normal, accepted behavior for the times? And how did this behavior, along with all the evil circumstance that ill-informed people associate with it, come to be known as sadism?

I am required to follow the path of sadism as it pertains to the medical field for a period of time, as this is where the origin of the word lies. There is probably a vast majority of people in the BDSM community who disagree with the word's definition as put forth in the medical literature. I will attempt to shed a favorable light on this subject by explaining the changes associated with the medical definition of sadism. It is my hope that you will agree, as evidenced by the changes made there, that it is no longer purely an evil sexual practice but can be an accepted sexual behavior.

Richard Freiherr von Krafft-Ebing, a German/Austrian psychiatrist who lived from 1840 to 1902, adopted the word "sadism" for professional use in 1898. However, in his work titled *Psychopathia Sexualis* written in 1886, he did discuss sadistic experiences as being sexual in nature.

"The experience of sexual, pleasurable sensations (including orgasm) produced by acts of cruelty, bodily punishment afflicted on one's person or when witnessed in others, be they animals or human beings. It may also consist of an innate desire to humiliate, hurt, wound or even destroy others in order, thereby, to create sexual pleasure in ones self." (p109)

By using the word "innate," Krafft-Ebing shows he firmly believes one can be born a sadist. I completely agree with this possibility, as I often say I am just wired this way. You will find later that behaviors classified as sadistic do not include the original proposal of sexual pleasure consequential to the watching of others receiving acts of cruelty or bodily punishment. This is especially important to me because I do become sexually aroused when watching a scene in which the bottom is suffering. Yet, I do not derive sexual pleasure while watching a fistfight or poking my patients with needles for blood draws. In addition, subsequent behavioral descriptors do not include animals.

Krafft-Ebing selected the word "sadism" to describe a set of sexual behaviors, specifically the behaviors enacted and written by the Marquis Donatien Alphonse Francois de Sade, a renowned French author who lived from 1740 to 1814. It is obvious the word "sadism" is derived from the name of de Sade himself. The original definition put forth did not mention the premise of either consensual or non-consensual acts. It can be argued that it addresses non-consensual behavior, as this is what the Marquis de Sade wrote about. The Marquis' works included graphic descriptions of acts in which the "victim" was made to suffer, feel pain, and be humiliated, which resulted in the sexual gratification of the aggressor. It is precisely the behavior of sexual gratification which was obtained from cruelty to another from which the word was derived. You may hear the term "sexual sadism." Given the fact that the word "sadism" was originated to explain a form of sexual gratification, many authorities believe it is redundant to say "sexual sadism" and simply say "sadism."

The Marquis de Sade's noted works include *120 Days of Sodom, Justine,* and *Juliette.*

> *He bleeds both of her arms and would have her remain standing while her blood flows; now and again he stops the bleeding and flogs her, then he opens the wounds again, and this continues until she collapses. He only discharges when she faints.* – 120 Days of Sodom

> *He attaches a girl to a St. Andrew's cross suspended in the air, and whips her with all his might, flaying her entire back. After which, he unties her and casts her out through a window, but mattresses are there to lighten her fall, upon hearing which he discharges.* – 120 Days of Sodom

> *She raises a storm, criticizing their behavior toward her and describing it as unjust. "Were it just," says the Duc, wiping his razor, "it would surely fail to give us an erection."* – 120 Days of Sodom

> *But the darling girl's pleas were worse than futile, for Dubourg, far from being disgusted by the spectacle of her suffering, actually savored it, delighted in it, thrived on it! Striking her once, twice, a third time, he fell madly on top of her and began nuzzling her bloody mouth.* – Justine

Not only did he write about acts of sexual perversion, it seems he indulged in such acts throughout his personal life, the most prominent being his involvement with Rose Keller. According to the court in which he was tried for his acts, the Marquis de Sade picked up Rose Keller and took her to a home in Arcueil where he reportedly bound and flogged her. It is not known if de Sade raped Rose Keller due to the lack of physical evidence.

Among the numerous reports of his participation in orgies, one well-known account states he hired four prostitutes to take part in one, which included a round of flogging. This is to say everyone got flogged including de Sade himself and his servant. It was this encounter for which the Marquis was arrested for poisoning and sodomy. It seems de Sade was accused of slipping something equivalent to Spanish fly into some aniseed sweets. Rather than sexually arousing the prostitutes, it made them very sick. Although, I have to wonder why you would have to give an aphrodisiac to a prostitute.

In 1898, Krafft-Ebing described this sadistic behavior as, "The quality of sadistic acts is defined by the relative potency of the tainted individual. If potent, the impulse of the sadist is directed to coitus, coupled with preparatory concomitant or consecutive maltreatment." Note how he describes the behavior of a sexual act being fueled by the "maltreatment" of another human. You should also see that he believes the amount of discomfort felt by the victim is a direct factor in the degree of sexual gratification. The psychiatric community then attached the classification and diagnostic criteria of "paraesthesia" to the sexual behavior.

The word "sadism" was originated to describe a behavior, not a psychological disorder. The classification and diagnostic criterion assigned to the behavior by the American Psychiatric Association (APA) are what make it a psychological disorder at times (in the United States). However, the classification and diagnostic criteria have been changed over the years by the APA; the behavior itself has not. If the behavior (sadism) is healthy, consensual, and not harmful to the person or others, it is not a disorder.

From 1886 till now, there really have been no changes in what sadistic behavior consists of. On the contrary, our view of what is healthy sadism and unhealthy sadism has changed.

I will now provide a time line for how the behavioral requirements have changed for the diagnosis of sexual sadism according to the APA as illustrated in the Diagnostic and Statistical Manual of Mental Disorders (DSM). Interjected will be my thoughts, as a sadist. I have skipped the DSM I (1952), II (1968) and III (1980) since sexual sadism was considered a mental disorder under any circumstances in those versions. By virtue of having sexually sadistic fantasies, one could be diagnosed with a mental illness; that's how bad it used to be.

DSM-III-Revision (1987) Sexual sadism – Over a period of at least six months, recurrent, intense sexually arousing fantasies, sexual urges, or behaviors involving acts (real, not simulated) in which the psychological or physical suffering (including humiliation) of the victim is sexually exciting to the person.

There is no mention of this being healthy when all parties involved are consenting. At this point still, all sexual sadism, according to the APA, is a disorder. This provides a basis to compare subsequent changes. The APA is the only reference I can find that still uses the term "sexual sadism." Once again, many authorities feel this is redundant.

DSM- IV 1994 – Sexual Sadism
A. Over a period of at least 6 months, recurrent, intense sexually arousing fantasies, sexual urges, or behaviors involving acts (real, not simulated) in which the psychological or physical suffering (including humiliation) of the victim is sexually exciting to the person.
B. The fantasies, sexual urges, or behaviors cause clinically significant distress or impairment in social, occupational, or other important areas of functioning.

Special attention should be drawn to paragraph "B" as the APA is trying to say that sexual sadism does not have to be a mental disorder. Both parts, A and B, must be present for the diagnosis of sexual sadism as a mental disorder. It's about damn time, and it only took them a hundred years from the inception of the word sadism to figure it out. Most certainly this description fits with the sexual habits written by the Marquis de Sade.

DSM-IV-Text Revision (2000) Sexual Sadism
A. Over a period of at least 6 months, recurrent, intense sexually arousing fantasies, sexual urges, or behaviors involving acts (real, not simulated) in which the psychological or physical suffering (including humiliation) of the victim is sexually exciting to the person.

B. The person has acted on these urges with a nonconsenting person, or the sexual urges or fantasies cause marked distress or interpersonal difficulty.

The APA explained the text revision for sexual sadism:

"Because some cases of Sexual Sadism may not involve harm to a victim (e.g., inflicting humiliation on a consenting partner), the wording for sexual sadism involves a hybrid of the DSM-III-R and DSM-IV wording (i.e., "the person has acted on these urges with a non-consenting person, or the urges, sexual fantasies, or behaviors cause marked distress or interpersonal difficulty").

Finally the APA realizes that people can and do engage in consensual sexual sadism. Healthy consensual sexual sadism does not fall into the realm of part "B." Nonetheless, some folks will throw out this standard definition on the basis of origin (the APA). This is why we sadists in the BDSM community attach the word "consensual" to make it consensual sadism. This describes the original basic behavior that the word was pulled from and modifies it to show it involves willing participants.

Currently the APA considers unhealthy sexual sadism a paraphilia – a psychosexual disorder which is comprised by thoughts, sexual fantasies, or acts with non-consenting people or objects involving pain or humiliation of oneself or another.

The World Health Organizations (WHO) endorses the International Statistical Classification of Diseases and Related Health Problems 10th Revision Version (ICD-10) for 2003, which has the following to say about sadism:

Disorders of adult personality and behaviour (F60-F69)
This block includes a variety of conditions and behaviour patterns of clinical significance which tend to be persistent and appear to be the expression of the individual's characteristic lifestyle and mode of relating to himself or herself and others. Some of these conditions and patterns of behaviour emerge early in the course of individual development, as a result of both constitutional factors and

social experience, while others are acquired later in life. Specific personality disorders (F60.-), mixed and other personality disorders (F61.-), and enduring personality changes (F62.-) are deeply ingrained and enduring behaviour patterns, manifesting as inflexible responses to a broad range of personal and social situations. They represent extreme or significant deviations from the way in which the average individual in a given culture perceives, thinks, feels and, particularly, relates to others. Such behaviour patterns tend to be stable and to encompass multiple domains of behaviour and psychological functioning. They are frequently, but not always, associated with various degrees of subjective distress and problems of social performance.

Under F65 – Disorders of sexual preference, Includes: paraphilias.
F65.5 Sadomasochism – A preference for sexual activity which involves the infliction of pain or humiliation, or bondage. If the subject prefers to be the recipient of such stimulation this is called masochism; if the provider, sadism. Often an individual obtains sexual excitement from both sadistic and masochistic activities. Masochism. Sadism.

I find it interesting that one must extract sadism from the term "sadomasochism." The deduction one must make is that, according to the ICD-10, sadism is a preference for sexual activity that involves the "provider" inflicting pain, humiliation or bondage. What is more compelling is how the ICD-10 pinpoints the activity of bondage. By denoting bondage, which is an activity that does not necessarily indicate pain or humiliation, the ICD-10 greatly deviates from other established definitions, such as the one adopted by the APA in DSM-IV-TR and those of the origin of the word sadism itself. It should also be scrutinized that bondage is only one of many activities that "…involves the infliction of pain or humiliation…" Nor is there an implication as to the severity of such bondage.

The "S" part of BDSM stands for both submission and sadism from what I have researched, although I have no idea who put the acronym together or how. However, we do know the origin of the word sadism and the context in which it was first used. Through the years of BDSM, this term has mutated into something it is not. So bastardized has it become from its definition of old, I was once told that, "I suppose you could argue that is not sadistic to give someone something they somehow enjoy, but in our world sadism tends to be more about who is delivering the pain, not about how it is received."

Yeah, sure, in some fairy tale world I guess. Why skew an established definition to make it fit you? I think for some strange reason, people wish to be identified as sadists. Maybe it is some "bad boy" image they think it gives them? Perhaps it makes them proud to be associated with this sexual minority?

There does not need to be, nor should there be, any modification required other than adding the word "consensual" to sadism in our world of BDSM. If you do not fit this behavior, don't change the established definition of a word, which describes a behavior, to fit you. Just call yourself a top.

Over the years I have heard many different definitions of what sadism really is. Often I am told that "my" definition does not match what "most" of the BDSM community views as sadism. But there is one difference between others and me here. A team of professionals, who in turn derived the definition from its origin, put forth "my" definition. So you see, it is not mine at all. I think you will find words like "pain," "cruelty," "suffering," or "hurting" in whatever definition of sadism you care to look up. People do not accept this fact.

Cambridge Dictionaries Online – "Sadism: the obtaining of pleasure, sometimes sexual, from being cruel to or hurting another person."

Dictionary.com – "1) Sadism: the deriving of sexual gratification or the tendency to derive sexual gratification from inflicting pain or emotional abuse on others. 2) The deriving of pleasure, or the tendency to derive pleasure, from cruelty. 3) Extreme cruelty."

Wikipedia Online Encyclopedia – "Sadism is the sexual pleasure or gratification in the infliction of pain and suffering upon another person."

I feel the Wikipedia definition most closely matches the original definition put forth for sadism. In my opinion, the Cambridge and Dictionary.com definitions miss the original behavior of sadism described by Krafft-Ebing, as they include pleasure from cruelty but not sexual pleasure. Some authorities in the medical and criminal fields do feel there is a difference between sadism and sexual sadism, and you see this reflected by the Cambridge characterization of "…pleasure, sometimes sexual…" Also note that it leaves out the word "pain" and appears to replace it with "hurting." In my travels I have had the opportunity to speak to many masochists – men and women who are sexually aroused by what others perceive as either physical or emotional pain. I have asked questions like, "So why don't you get sexually stimulated when you stub a toe?" "Because it hurts."

The Cambridge and Dictionary.com definitions include an area of specialization that the Wikipedia definition does not, which is the possibility of cruelty without sexual gratification. I often use the example of a person who kicks the family pet because it makes them happy, not sexually aroused; this is not a sadist but simply a person who is mean and cruel.

Pain, as defined, is an unpleasant sensation as a result of trauma, disease, or an emotional disorder; suffering, or distress. This to me implies that a person who feels pain is not happy about it. For example, having dental work is painful for most of us, although I am sure there are a few people out there who may like the sensations of dental work. Note how I changed the word "pain" to "sensation."

We feel sensations when our senses are stimulated; we then have perceptions of the stimulus. Thus they are highly individual and idiosyncratic to each of us. They can be interpreted into many different categories, if you will. Some sensations can be pleasurable while others can be unpleasant. When we define pain, it is an unpleasant sensation; hence people go to great lengths in pain clinics not to feel it. Pain hurts people.

I have said it before and I will say it again – a masochist is a sadist's worst enemy. I do say this a bit tongue in cheek to get people to really think about what "painful" sensations are like for a masochist. When we look at a masochist, they ultimately interpret what the rest of us would identify as pain, as pleasure. What others perceive as negative, they interpret as positive. Thus, it is not pain to them.

You see, masochists do feel and interpret some sensations as painful, as hurting. Pain is only pain when the person receiving it interprets it as a negative, unpleasant or suffering sensation. I may think I am causing another pain because, well — damn — it sure looks like it would hurt *me*. But in reality, they enjoy the sensation and feel it is a positive one. The sensation that is taking place does not hurt them.

This brings to mind my recent tattoo work. While speaking with my tattoo artist, he told me that many times he has to stop and give people a break because it hurts them too much. This applies to all areas of the body that he has worked with. While getting work done on the base of my neck I started to laugh because it tickled. It held up his work because I had to settle myself down and hold still. But he told me for other people it is a very painful place to tattoo.

While we may hate labels, definitions, and language, they are important for communication and general understanding. I think after looking at the definition of sadism, the interpretation and perception of what a bottom is receiving is very vital, particularly to a sadist.

To gain current understanding of how BDSM people view sadism, I started an online discussion in January of 2006. While reading the rest of this chapter you will find various quotes from what was posted. I learned in this discussion how much some have distanced themselves from the origins of sadism. Below are a couple comments referring to BDSM; Risk-Aware Consensual Kink (RACK); Safe, Sane, and Consensual (SSC); and sadism.

> *"One is to recruit new members and another is to make people feel comfortable once they get here. As a result sexual sadism is often divorced from its literal meaning – dictionary or DSM – even when that's what those who are using the term wish to communicate."* – mike bond

"But in a Scene where every act has 'play' attached to it, it's hard to take assertions of sexual sadism literally." – mike bond

People do recruit into the lifestyle. We bring in new people fresh out of their closets and make them feel comfortable with words like "play" and "toys." Acronyms like SSC and RACK make newbies feel safe from harm, I guess. I really take exception to the words "play" and "toys" incidentally. At one time it was called "working a boy over." What we used were tools, not toys.

So here we have the preprogrammed recruit "SSC sadistic top" using "toys" in a "play" session at a public BDSM event. Then they look over and see what some may call a "real" consensual sadist and their bottom does not look like they are enjoying what is being done to them. Their partner is even saying, "No, stop!" *Holy bat droppings, Batman!!! This must be non-consensual and unsafe. Get a DM quick, as this scene must be stopped.* Do you see how not giving the full picture of sadism can be harmful to our community?

It was during this online discussion that I really learned there is a vast amount of misconceptions about sadism. Or at least there were many opinions. What I am about to say may be offensive to some, but I feel that it is true. It is conceivable that some of the people who posted comments have never had a BDSM sexual encounter, let alone a run-in with a sadist. I affectionately call these people "armchair" tops and bottoms. *But FifthAngel, what about the folks who are scared to come out of the closest and act on their sexual fantasies in real life?* The hardcore philosophy is, "Get over it and get on with it."

There are people better suited than I to help newbies realize who they are when just coming out of the vanilla world. I have been taught and abide under less gentle beliefs; thus, I do not coddle newbies as much as others might. I say tell them the truth about consensual sadism and the origins of the word. Teach them about what they will see if they venture into the world of "public" BDSM.

I will admit that I am not the best educator for every subject in BDSM. I do cater to the more extreme side of the lifestyle, as this is who I am and what I best relate to. Often I am recruited to teach the edgier side of sadism. As a result of this, I mostly deal with experienced Scene people.

But I can't tell you where people have gotten the notions that I am about to share with you. I have to consider that some of it is personal opinion with no factual basis whatsoever. Or is it that this is what people want to believe for whatever reason and reject our roots?

> *"You have raised an interesting point. If a sadist is someone who is aroused by inflicting pain on another, it should not matter if that person does not care if the masochist is experiencing pleasure or suffering as a result of the pain."* – Kelly aka Teach

This goes back to what sadism is and the misinterpretation of the pain a person is believed to be feeling. Pain does not cause the sensation of pleasure in anyone or else it would not be called pain.

I will interject a theory here. Some scientists believe pain and pleasure are on the same continuum as the mind interprets a sensation. For example, a sensation like caning the feet may feel pleasurable at first, but eventually the stimulus will become painful if done long enough or hard enough. The masochist would become sexually aroused from a caning in the pleasurable range, yet feel pain from the same activity further down the road. Again, the sensations we are talking about would be painful to others. Don't try to throw in tickling with a feather here.

> *"If a sadist gets off on torturing another person and a sexual masochist gets off on being tortured, it almost seems like you're saying that if a sexual masochist is getting off then it is somehow less of an experience for the sadist."* – Laurie

Quick, go back to page 17 and read the passage I quoted from de Sade's writing concerning the Duc. My online reply to this was, "Um, yea…that is what sexual sadism is."

> *"I see what you're saying about how the sadist should be the one who's getting off, but I think there is a flip side...this is after all*

consensual BDSM. If you didn't have a willing partner, it would be a criminal activity, so there must be some intrinsic pleasure for the masochist." – Laurie

I never mentioned non-consensual sadism. I threw out the DSM definition and some people jumped to the conclusion that unpleasant sensations could not be consented to. Some feel that there are only sexual masochists in this lifestyle, but there are people who want to feel pain for the sake of feeling pain. They have a need to be beat to catharsis. They want to cry and purge by suffering to learn about themselves.

Also, we as sadists know you are getting something from letting us hurt you. We are not so stupid to think you get nothing from it. In the moment, those who subject themselves to sadists are in real pain and would rather be someplace else. That does not mean they don't later masturbate to the memory of the encounter. It could be that it is an act of service; we will read about this later. In such cases, the individual will endure pain because they take pleasure in knowing they make the sadist happy.

As a sadist, it makes me happy to know that the encounter was pleasurable, at some point, for my partner. Yes, they were really hurting and hating me in the moment, which makes me cum, but they are happy after it is over. I do not think anyone would consent to a sadist if they got nothing from it.

> *"Secondly, I personally prefer to engage in sadistic mind-fucking and if that then coincidentally leads to physically fucking then all the better, but the latter has nothing to do with being a sadist."*
> – Kindred

This person's acts are solely mean and not sadistic in nature. I remind you of the definition which mentioned, "The obtaining of pleasure, sometimes sexual, from being cruel to…." I sense this person does not connect cruelty and sexual pleasure since they don't care if they get fucked after mind-fucking another. They are not mind-fucking to get sexually aroused. The simple fact is that not every person who causes the sensation of "pain" (either emotional or physical) does it for sexual reasons. I can assure you there are many folks like this in the BDSM community as I have seen and spoken to them in my classes and abroad.

Some fail to understand why it's not the same for a sadist working on a masochist who enjoys the pain. They wonder how a sadist could possibly find a willing partner who submits to painful activities they don't enjoy, and they wonder when this becomes abusive.

This always makes me chuckle a little because I am a known sadist and I have no problems getting people to let me do unpleasant stuff to them. Shoot, I always tell people up front what I am by giving "my" definition of what sadism is, and they still want to give it a go. Also, I will say this once so remember it well: it becomes abuse when the person no longer consents to the pain. Later there will be more about consent and the use of "safewords" and those who choose not to use them.

Others speak of the pain needing to be consensual in order to avoid abuse. They believe the bottom's pleasure must be important to the sadist because the two must have a relationship that extends beyond their BDSM scenes.

Are they saying that, by the definition I provided, they speculate pain could not be consented to? Hell, even the APA says you can consent to pain and suffering. It depends on what is negotiated whether the sadist is to be concerned with the pleasure of the partner at any point in the scene. There are scenes that I have done that the bottom will do for the sake of suffering pain. They are not interested in feeling anything pleasurable in the moment. Can I get off sexually by this? Hell, yeah! It gives me one less thing to worry about. (I laughed to myself as I wrote that.)

I don't want you thinking that I disagreed with everything that was posted in that discussion. There were some people who really understood what sadism was and still should be about. I say "still" because there is no good reason for us to distance ourselves from our roots. What the Marquis de Sade wrote about were primarily non-consensual acts. These are not the roots that I am talking about. I am talking about pure, hot, sexually charged consensual sadism where your partner agrees to feel pain because it gets you off.

I disagree with all "tops" being grouped together as sadists by virtue of the fact that they all create sensations for their partners. The truth is that not all tops are sadists, and you just read my proof. So here are the words of the people who I think have accepted who they are and what makes them happy – the sadists and the people who let them do mean things:

> *"My bottoms pleasure and/or comfort is not My concern when we go there. As a matter of fact, it pleases me most when my boi is taking more than could possibly be 'enjoyable.' And yes, the excitement, the power and the energy does occasionally end in orgasm for me...if not 'in the moment' then shortly afterward."*
> -Ms. Cindy

> *"Absolutely. my own slave endures the pain inflicted by needles and cutting not because she enjoys it but because she knows that it gives me pleasure. Regardless of the fact that she finds no pleasure in it I do. I get excited. turned on. I ride the energy of her pain and suffering until I orgasm and beyond. Is it consensual? Yes. Is she having 'fun'? No."* – name withheld by request

> *"As the 's' side of a D/s relationship, I know that my Mistress quite enjoys a number of pain related activities that don't turn me on. I consent to and accept that there are times when we will engage in these activities. I know that engaging in them will not cause me permanent harm, however I know that my Mistress is very turned on by the activity, my reaction to the activity etc."*
> – name withheld by request

> *"She is not asking me to do things that are non-consensual, and we have built up a trust relationship that provides me with the knowledge that she will not do me permanent harm, or render me unable to do my sports or work etc. She is asking me to engage in activities that I don't like.... to accept types of pain that does not turn me on, that I don't want and she is asking me to do this because it turns her on, so I submit. It is for her pleasure, not mine. I do not see this as abuse."* – name withheld by request

And whoever said that a consensual sadist wants to permanently harm people? You can bet bottoms that I have sessions with feel unpleasant pain and hurting. But that does not mean they are all permanently damaged. Sadism can be performed in a safe environment.

Why is any of this a concern? The psychological effects consensual sadists can have on the bottoms they "play" with can be devastating if there are misunderstandings. Say a bottom has done scenes with tops who only inflicted sensations that the bottom liked, but those tops called themselves sadists. Now the consensual sadist starts to create unpleasant sensations for the bottom because that is what a consensual sadist does. The inexperienced and poorly educated bottom freaks. This does not do any good for the consensual sadist either, to have a bottom react poorly. Who knows where it could go from there.

If nothing more comes from this book and this chapter other than that we should learn to communicate better as sadists what our needs are, I would be overjoyed. For the bottoms, if a person says he or she is a sadist, ask what that means to them. Because there are very different opinions of what sadism really is these days, we must learn to talk to one another in plain simple terms and make sure they are understood. When someone asks what I mean when I say I am a sadist, I tell them, "I want to make you feel unpleasant sensations from which I will get sexual gratification when you dislike what I do." If you don't want to create unpleasant sensations, call yourself a top.

One Sick Puppy

Ever have random thoughts of hitting another person, raping another, or cutting someone open to feel their heart beating in your hand? Or perhaps you fantasize about bathing in the blood of your loved one? So what's stopping you, besides a jail sentence, potential hospital bill, or just plain common sense?

Again, what separates me from the serial-killer-type sadist is that what I do is consensual. However, since the dead can't suffer, serial killers who perform post-mortem sexual acts are not sadists but just people who are cruel to others. My partners give me permission to do whatever it is I do. Thank goodness I am not alone in my fantasies. Not that it would matter, though. Often in my classes about gun scenes, I ask if anyone ever had the desire to kill another because they found it sexually exciting. In each class, people have raised hands. Does that make them mentally disturbed? No, because they have not acted on it, I hope. To have fantasies is one thing. To plan, calculate, and act on them is another.

More widespread is the fantasy to bathe in another's blood. By the attendance in my classes about blood scenes, this is something common to BDSM folks and very doable without a life-in-prison consequence. Also, I think this is a more prevalent urge than most are willing to admit out loud. But how do you tell your partner you want to smear their blood all over them and yourself and then fuck them?

In perhaps what many would consider extreme scenes, I live out my sadistic fantasies. Such images and random thoughts enter my mind throughout everyday life. Be it driving to the climbing gym or watching a movie at the theater, my mind gets stimulated with ideas of sexually sadistic scenes. But there is a time and place for everything.

While having dinner with my slave in a restaurant, I closed my eyes. When I opened them, before me was my slave with hooks in her flesh. Attached to the hooks were chains going in all directions. The image of the chains and hooks was like an overlay of reality. But would this image be something I could duplicate? Sure, I could put the hooks in, but would it be safe? There was no question that she would be willing to do it. So began the logistical planning.

Hooks and chain can always be found in my home dungeon. The difficult part would be finding a piece of equipment that would provide overhead attachment points as well as attachment points in all directions around her body. Ideally something similar to a cage would work, but I would need to add attachment points. Also, I needed a cage tall enough to stand in that had about 3-4 feet of access on all sides.

Long ago I learned never to be in a hurry when working out my fantasies. I was confident the equipment I needed would turn up in time. So as I traveled with my slave over the next few months, my hooks and chains went with me. Entering every new dungeon, my normal walk around inspecting equipment became ritual. Then, at the Camp Crucible event in 2005, I found what I was searching for. The piece of equipment looked like a four-legged bug without the body. Black in color, each leg had welded attachment rings spaced about three feet apart, beginning at the floor and continuing up each leg to the top, where all four legs united.

Our good friend Barbara Nitke was attending Camp that year and asked what I would be up to, so I explained to her what I was intending to do. Immediately she asked if she could photograph the scene. My reply was, "Sure." I was going to ask her to anyway. Barbara has photographed us many times before, so we know how each other works. Barbara becomes part of my scenes: at times she becomes so absorbed that I have no idea where she is or even how close she gets. Other times, when she actually does say something to a bystander, hers is the only other voice I hear.

On the trip, I brought hooks ranging from 18 gauge to 12 gauge, and chain of various sizes and weight. As scenes like this typically go for me, I asked my slave to leave so I might prepare the area. I sat in front of the equipment and closed my eyes to place the image of the scene in my mind. One thing that I had done was put the equipment into a corner, which is always my preferred place to scene in a public dungeon. This eliminates any potential traffic flow through the area. That way, if people chose to watch, the scene would be blocked in.

Barbara was wandering about the dungeon shooting different scenes. She knew where I was, so when the scene began she could come and go as she pleased.

My slave had an idea of what I wanted to do, but lacked the complete details of what was in my mind. She had explained to me she was a bit nervous and did not know if she could take what I had in mind. But I knew that once I began she would be fine.

My slave's name, given to her by me, is "angel in chains." She earned this name as part of her collaring ceremony. In the past, I have placed needles or staples in her back and attached light chains to them, running the other ends of the chains to piercings or staples in the backs of her hands, thus giving her wings of chain.

I knew if I duplicated her wings again, she would be in the proper mindset for what I needed to do. But this time, the chain would be much heavier and the attachment points in her back would be eight 12-gauge hooks.

My slave was facing outward towards the rest of the dungeon space. I had her stand in the middle of the four-legged bug — then a new image flooded my mind like a pail of red paint thrown against a white wall. After all the hooks were placed, I would bleed her. In my mind, blood was dripping from her body. Shooting the full length of her white skin, it pooled on the floor.

To insert the needles for hook setting, I had her kneel down and lean forward. Soon all eight hooks were set in her back, and I began to attach the heavy chain. A while back, in my own dungeon, I had laid out the chains and fixed them at the proper lengths. The equipment had attachment points at about shoulder height, which was perfect. Her wings would remain attached whether she was standing or kneeling, which would later be a remarkable unplanned addition to the scene's eroticism. She was now in the proper mindset. The additional weight of the chain intensified the sensation of the hook placements.

I had her stand in the center of the frame; then I began to set the other hooks. Soon, there were chains jutting out in all directions. Up, down, sideways, and crossing – I had every angle of movement controlled. There was not one direction she could move without feeling tension on the hooks. While placing hooks and needles, I never count how many I place because it is not about numbers. Later, an observer told me she had 22 hooks in her – he had counted as the scene went along.

Soon, everything was where I wanted it. Barbara had been taking photos off and on, but apparently she had left after all of the hooks and chains were placed. Now it was time for a blood bath. To say my slave has a fetish for blood is an understatement. She gets blood on her and she goes to la-la land. Torture for her is my bleeding her and not allowing her to lick it off.

I began to poke holes in her veins – that gets you far more blood than a cutting. I accessed veins in her arms and neck. Her external jugular veins received multiple holes on both sides of her neck. These are large veins and carry a large amount of blood. Also, the blood from her neck would drip all the way down her breasts, torso, and legs to pool at her feet.

Then I heard Barbara's voice, "Geez, I can't leave for a minute." Soon came the flash of a camera. I smiled to myself. When Barbara had left, my slave was clean, not a drop of blood on her, just bound with hooks and chains. When Barbara returned, she was covered in blood from head to toe. Quite the change for Barbara, I guess.

Perhaps I should have mentioned that my cock was hard all the while. Now I wanted to fuck my slave – yes, with her covered in blood with hooks and chains holding her in place. No, I am not talking about a nice love-making session. My cock was hard and I needed to fuck her hard and painfully. But hell, she was standing up, immobilized, with sharp thingies sticking out of her everywhere. I would get poked. We are fluid bonded, so it would not pose a threat of disease transmission, but it might hurt, damn it.

Oh wait, she can kneel with her wings still attached. Doggie-style is a favorite position of mine. It allows deep penetration and hurts her when I pound her cervix with my cock. Not to mention that hitting her cervix with the head of my cock gives me a great deal of stimulation. So I began to remove some hooks. I thought to myself, "Does she think the scene is ending?" I did not tell her what I was going to do.

All the hooks were removed except the eight 12-gauge ones running the full length of her well-defined, muscular back. She began to bleed from the holes where the other hooks had been, which further fueled my sadism. I had to be inside her.

Positioning my slave on her knees and myself behind her, I removed my hakama and shoved her forward. Suddenly, she cried out in pain. But my cock was not inside her yet – the hooks in her back were being pulled. As I propelled her forward, it jerked on the hooks because of the equipment's positioning. The attachment points were now above and behind her. My reality was far superior to the images that had entered my mind months ago.

I began to fuck her from behind while placing my hands on her hips to control her every movement. Each time I shoved her hips forward, it pulled on her wings, causing more sensation. Each time I pulled her hips back to me, my cock pounded her cervix. Soon ecstasy overrode my mind, body, and soul. I grabbed her wings in each hand. No longer would I pull her hips back with my hands. I yanked her back onto my cock by pulling on the hooks and chains, only to force her forward again by ramming my cock deeper into her.

Intermittently, I would reach forward to feel the blood continuing to drip from her breasts, neck, and arms. A few times I had leaned against her, getting poked by the hooks myself. Soon I had blood on my body as well, while we were fucking in the public dungeon.

I have no idea how long that scene was; it did not matter whether it was thirty minutes or two hours. Nor do I know how many were watching. We lay exhausted for a few minutes with her wings still attached. I reached up to release her wings from the attachment points on the equipment, and then placed the tips over her shoulders to shroud her in the chains. I knew she was smiling and feeling an overwhelming sense of love and security. She held her wings as I removed the last remaining hooks. Each hook I pulled out resulted in more bloodshed. I sat and watched the blood run down her back. Soon, I was licking the blood from her.

As we slowly returned to reality, I began to notice people once again. Some were sitting in chairs while others lay on the floor watching. Some were smiling and others were crying. I was later told the crying was due to the love, energy, and passion they had witnessed between my slave and me.

For some, this may sound like fiction out of some one-handed novel. For me, it is but one fantasy that entered my mind to later become reality. While mild to some within the lifestyle, the average man on the street would have no comprehension of how I could even imagine such a thing. But that is how my mind works. It is a free flow of images and thoughts. While my slave may have wanted to be someplace else during the pain, I promise you she has masturbated and orgasmed with images of that scene in her head. So that makes one more sick puppy, I would guess.

But just as one person's terrorist is another's revolutionary, one person's sexual urges can be another's nightmare. It would seem I am not alone, though. As sick and twisted as it may seem to an outsider to see a woman drenched in blood with hooks in her back being painfully fucked, people were compelled to stay and witness such events at 2 am in a public dungeon.

Other things that may fit into the sick puppy category include mouth suturing, eye suturing, gun scenes, naso-gastric tubes, rape scenes, and such. There are, however, some very heavy body modification folks out there who practice slicing open testicles, tongue splitting, and so forth. But they, to my understanding, do not do it to get off sexually. Some may, and if so, they are sicker puppies than I am. But it's all good.

What Are You Thinking?

I am often asked what I think about when I am inflicting pain on another human being. At times, I think of nothing, while other times I think of, well, sex. For a sadist, that is what it is about, after all. But for the sake of my curious readers, I will go into further detail.

Perhaps I should tell you that I don't consider what I do with my slave "play" or a "scene;" rather, it is just sex to me. I mean, I don't set up my home dungeon for a scene. It gets set up to have sex. Sure there are times when there is no actual intercourse, but those times are more about teaching.

The most memorable sex sessions are those that happen spontaneously. There is a certain luxury to having a 24/7 live-in slave who does not say no to sex. I am spoiled in that I can be sitting watching television and get inspired to have sex and have it in a matter of moments. Spontaneous, uninhibited sex is the best, in my personal opinion. To act on instinct is a very primal part of us. This brings me to my first story about what I think about during sex.

I was laying in my bed one afternoon, taking a siesta with my slave. I must have had some erotic dream because I woke up horny as hell. I pounced on my slave. Now I will be the first to tell you I never listened to my mother when she told me not to bite. I am a biter – always have been, always will be.

So I woke, pounced on the slave and began biting her breasts, nipples, arms, anything that got in my way. When I bite, it is very hard and causes a great deal of pain. Over the years I have learned how hard I can bite without breaking the skin. The skill lies in which teeth you bite with.

There I was chewing on her flesh when an image of the African plain flashed into my mind. At that point, some people would stop and wonder, "What the heck am I thinking?" I just let images and thoughts flow freely. Next came images of lions feasting on the carcass of a zebra. Suddenly, I was among them feeding on my prey.

I could feel the meat and bone being crushed between my jaws. Then the carcass began to be pulled away from me. I pulled back. I was hungry and nobody was going to take my food away. It was a fresh kill, and as my teeth clenched down harder, I could feel the blood squirting and dripping down my face. The tug of war continued.

It was a fight for survival and I had to win. If I did not feed, I would starve. So I began to pull and tug at the flesh of the zebra. Twisting my head, snarling and growling, I pulled my prey away from my competitors. Soon my meal was being dragged across the desert floor.

It was then that I heard my slave's voice: "Master, please look at me. I need to see your eyes." There was fear in her voice. Doing my best to continue, I am sure I did not understand her at first and she repeated her words.

Opening my eyes and thoughts to the present, I realized I was gnawing on her stomach while I was attempting to drag her across the bed, using just my teeth. She had felt I was not in my own mind – that I was not thinking of her as human, and it concerned her. My cock was so hard at this point, the break to reality made it painful.

Flipping my slave over to her stomach resulted in the flooding of new images. No longer the carcass of a zebra, she was now a lioness being forced into the dirt. I needed to spread my seed and build upon the pride. Instinctively, she resisted. Using my paws, I moved her hair and bit her hard on the back of the neck and shoved my cock hard as far as it would go. There were no thoughts of using lube or concerns if it would hurt her.

Occasionally, I would release my grip on her neck only to drag my claws down her back. Still suffering from my cock being so hard, I fucked her as hard and deep as I could. I remember biting her neck one last time in preparation for the release of my pain. Then the pain was gone, and I lay on top of her, not supporting any of my weight myself; I was happy looking down at my sweat- and saliva-covered slave.

In the above story, the pain was incidental, not intentional. At first I was fighting for food, then later I needed another cub to continue my lineage. The pain my slave felt was a result of primal instinct that happens every day in the animal kingdom. Does this imply that many species of animals are sexually sadistic? I hope not; it is just the way they are, which is how many humans are, if we allow ourselves to be – if we give ourselves permission.

While it may seem we are not in touch with reality and are out of our minds, some may wonder how we do not harm one another. In primal states, I believe that in another part of the subconscious mind we know just how much pain we may be causing and are aware of the physical well-being of our partner. Over the years, never once have I caused my slave to require medical attention. Never once has my biting resulted in bloodshed.

Let me take a break from telling what I think about when I am a sadist and tell you what I *don't* think about.

I don't think about how well I am doing something. While flogging, for example, I am not thinking about my technique, nor do I think about whether they like it or not. So what if they like a thuddy flogger and I am using a stingy one? Who cares if they are crying? That is just a sign of either suffering or release: both are good. I don't consciously think about not harming someone. I am confident in my skills to instinctively know how hard to hit someone.

Probably, first and most important, I don't care who is watching and if they understand what goes on between my partners and myself.

I do, however, prep dungeon monitors when I scene in public. I feel this is common courtesy and just plain common sense. To my credit and justification, never once have I had a scene stopped. But then again, it could be that I wield a four-foot-long sword. No matter, give people a rough idea that you scene hard and that "no" does not mean "no."

People worry about others watching. "Am I good enough to flog in public?" "What if I make a mistake and wrap?" "What if they think I am being too hard?"

Let me assure you that "mistakes" happen to everyone, even me. I will throw in some unsolicited advice here. Never flog with your shirt off if you sweat a lot. While flogging a boy in a public dungeon, the flails of my flogger stuck to my sweaty back. As fate would have it, my hand continued forward. The flogger flails got unstuck as I lost my grip, propelling the flogger through the air, and whacking the boy in the back of the head with the wooden handle. The flogger bounced off the boy's head and into a large mirror in front of us. Luckily, the mirror did not break. Without thinking, I began to flog with the one remaining flogger. The boy had no issue; the mirror was fine; why stop the energy?

But if I would have freaked out that I screwed up in a public scene, it would have made the entire dungeon aware and would have stopped the scene. As the saying goes, "Shit happens." This is not to say that I don't care, no matter what happens.

I don't think about the pain my partners are in. They feel pain. They feel suffering. I know their pain and suffering will end. As a former emergency room nurse and current critical care nurse, I learned to detach from my emotions early in my career. My detaching began even before that with my martial arts training.

In martial arts, my fellow students became my friends. Some were friends even before we started to train together. When it came to sparring, we had to set aside friendship. Training with the mindset that four enemies are attacking you, room for friendship only gets you hurt, even killed. You practice with the intent to harm if you have to. You have to fight your friends to learn to fight your enemies.

With nursing in the emergency and critical care areas, emotions and caring too much can lead to more death. Let's say I have been caring for a patient in my ICU for six weeks straight. Over the course of these six weeks I have learned the names of all their close family members, seen pictures of grandchildren, and even received an occasional "thank you" lunch from the family. Then the patient dies. Yes, I feel sad and may even cry with the family. An hour later I am wrapping the patient in a plastic shroud to be placed in a refrigerator.

Another nurse has been watching my other critically ill patient. I am still emotionally upset from my first patient dying as I resume care. As a result of my mental state, mistakes begin to happen. Medication errors, miscalculations, and forgetfulness consume me. One mistake leads to another as I become more flustered and emotionally upset. The final result could be my mistakes harming my other patient. Has this ever happened to me? No. But I have seen nurses' emotions over death leave room for mistakes. It is a good thing that other nurses were present to catch those mistakes before they harmed a patient.

So have I been trained to detach from emotions to reach a goal? Yes, I was taught from a young age to do just that. Do I think that had influence over my becoming a sadist? No, but it is a useful skill to detach from emotions at times.

There was one time that I allowed myself to feel another's pain in a scene. I had been using my sais and shinai on my slave to the point that she was in a state of unconsciousness – meaning I inflicted pain on her and her body did not respond. Her breathing and pulse were fine; it's just that her mind was in another place – not unlike my state of mind when I was in the African plains. Peering down at her as I hovered over her body, I opened my mind and heart to feel. Pain consumed me. I felt all the agony she had endured prior to entering an altered state. Pain hurts, even if it is temporary. Emotional pain, I believe, is worse than physical pain. I began to cry. My tears falling down my face landed upon her chest. My slave's own eyes filled with tears as she peered up at me in a state of confusion. She became frightened, not knowing what was wrong or why I was crying. Cradling my face in her hands, she began to cry even more. Never before had she seen me cry during a scene. Never before had I attempted to feel another's pain while being a sadist.

It was not about sex at that point. I had walked her path of pain. I understood from her side what she had endured to get where she was. I had always known what it was like for me to endure pain, but never another.

In the simplest terms, though, I still think about nothing intentional for the most part. Later in this book you will read essays from my slave and other friends who have been on the receiving end of my sadism, as well as spiritual journeys they took.

My partners will speak of their thoughts, reactions, and such. I will enlighten you as to what I think of during these events. Long have I known that pain and extreme sensations can lead to altered states of being. I know that because I have been there myself. Because I know what is on the other side, I do what I do to help others learn about themselves.

I do not look at myself as a healer, a shaman, or a spiritual leader, although others have called me just that. We all have different abilities, skills, and gifts. While I could not grow plants to save my life, I am damn good at poking needles in people both professionally and for fun. As a result of my ability to kill living foliage, I have silk flowers and plants around my house. Because I am good with needles, I have hundreds of needles and hooks as well as suspension gear in my dungeon. But why poke needles in people when it is not about sex?

I am a teacher of life, I guess, granted the skills to help people look at life in a different way. Name it a calling if you want, but I feel compelled to teach and share what I have been given.

As I placed six 8-gauge needles into Travis Wilson's back, I knew it hurt. Hell, I could hear that it hurt. It hurt as each hook was placed – up until the last one. Then there was no pain for him.

While putting the needles through his flesh, I thought about where he could go once suspended from hooks. My focus was not on his pain, but his journey. Every ounce of skill and care I possess goes into setting each hook. In this realm, it is not about wanting to cause pain to get off. It comes with the territory – the pain, that is.

The interesting part is that I have a choice to turn it into sexual energy. The first time I performed a hook suspension on my slave, I wanted to have sex while she was dangling from my ceiling. There I was, looking at my slave hanging in the middle of the air and then suddenly my cock started to tingle and I wanted to fuck her.

"What are you, sick or something? She is in on a spiritual journey, you jerk."

"Get those thoughts out of here, you sick bastard."

"Maybe next time."

So I shut down my sadist element for the sake of her journey. So you see, it is not always about me getting my rocks off.

There are times when random thoughts enter my mind; it is only natural. It is how I am wired. But sometimes the moral and ethical thing to do is to override them. Could I have let the pain Travis felt feed my sexual urges? Most certainly. But it would have been inappropriate.

The same goes for other cathartic scenes that I have had. The focus becomes the journey, not the sex, not my inflicting pain I know they can't stand. Whether it be flogging, punching, kicking, caning, or hooks, the concern is where the bottom is going. Pain is how they get there.

Remember this and you will care enough to inflict the very best.

The Lighter Side of SM

So you may be thinking that me being a sadist is all about me beating some poor, manipulated bottom until they cry and I cum. I hate to burst your bubble, but it can also be fun. The lighter side of sadism can be just as erotic to me as suturing a bottom's mouth closed. Following is an essay I wrote a number of years ago to explain how sadism can play a large part in a dominant/submissive relationship's everyday activities.

Masterism vs. Sadism

We all know what sadism is, but you may be wondering what the heck is "Masterism." Well you won't find it in any English dictionary, or even a Bondage, Discipline, and SadoMasochism (BDSM) dictionary for that matter.

An "ism" is a theory or system. Thus Masterism is the theory of Mastering slaves as it pertains to BDSM. Master-ism is a term that I made up to differentiate between what Masters do and what sadists do.

We all agree there is a vast array of Master/slave (M/s) dynamics. The one I wish to address is the M/s relationship with the Master also being a sadist.

While driving down a road one evening, my slave, slave leslie, turned to me and asked why I made things so difficult sometimes. I gathered my thoughts for a moment and replied:

"It's my job as a Master to teach you how to serve me; it's my job as a sadist to completely screw that up."

She had a blank look on her face for an instant then pulled out a pen and paper and began to write. I asked her what she was doing, to which she replied, "I am writing that down so I don't forget."

She realized that there is a huge difference between Masterism and Sadism. Please let me give you an example of the disparities.

Masterism – I trained my slave not to eat without permission.

Sadism – I find ways to trick my slave into eating without permission.

Once, I held food in front of her mouth. She gave me a puppy dog look: "Is it okay?" I raised my eyebrows as if to say, "Yes." She opened her mouth, I placed the food in it, and she began to chew. Ah ha — busted!

But I am a nice Master, having told her, "Go by the last given verbal order." (Key word here being "verbal.")

Thus it has become increasingly difficult for me to ensnare her in my traps. But never fear; I have the mind of a sadist.
Another example:

Masterism – I grant you the privilege of being identified as my slave.

Sadism – I will trick you into thinking you have this privilege before you officially do just to see if I can "catch" you.
The family name of my slave is "angel in chains" which she earned through rite of passage with me. I decided to make her community name "slave leslie."

In an evil Sadism trick hidden behind Masterism, I wrote "slave leslie" on a sticky note and handed it to her. I even went into her Black Rose 2002 profile and changed her identification badge to read "slave leslie."

Mind now, I had said nothing verbally about the name change

so she did not have permission to use "slave leslie."

While testing the email boxes for our web site, she sent an email to my address and signed it "slave leslie." Damn, I am good! Well, as a sadist and plotting schemer, that is. She fell right into my ambush.

Please understand: I do not impose any punishment with these traps. Well, there was one time when I made her eat with her fingers after she looked at me for permission and I replied, "Duh." It must be noted that "Duh" does not mean "You may eat."

It is for my own amusement as a sadist that I create these situations. The reminder that she must always be alert because she has a Master who is a sadist and will screw with her head any chance he gets is sufficient punishment.

At times my slave will get down on herself for "always screwing up." Well, it is the job of a sadist to ensure that happens. It would be my recommendation to slaves who serve under a combination of Masterism and Sadism not to take to heart the amusement that we inflict. There is no such thing as a "perfect" slave when your Master is a sadist.

By constantly changing what we want, we can confuse and frustrate another. Sadism can be broken down into two areas: physical and emotional. Physical sadism will eventually lead to emotional sadism as the bottom begins to dislike the pain you are causing. More about that later. Here I wish to talk about the playful side of sadistic foreplay.

It just tickles my butt to see my slave get all flustered and stomp her foot. I can always tell when I have gotten to her; she makes this certain face that causes her mouth to take on an odd shape. She also makes the same face when she knows I am right and she is wrong.

Being who I am, I am always messing with people's heads in a fun way. Once I was teaching a class titled: "The Ultimate Guide to Being a Lazy Top." Another female was helping with the class. To fit the theme of the class, they brought in an authentic La-Z-Boy™ chair. I taught the entire class sitting in the chair. My assistant handed me a cup of cashews and Goldfish™. I was not in the mood for Goldfish, so I asked her to take them out. Truth be told, I just needed a reason to mess with her.

So she sorted through the cup, taking out each orange cracker, and handed the cup back to me. "You missed one." I handed the cup back to her. Eventually she dumped the contents of the cup onto a table and discovered there were no remaining Goldfish in the cup. Correct — I had lied.

But she looked so cute sitting there on the floor searching for the invisible piece of cracker. I am sure she knew that I had lied. But she was going to make every attempt to ensure that she did what she was told. Why would a person subject herself to such meaningless torture? I offer this in my defense: It teaches them patience.

I am convinced that my martial arts teachers were just mean and maybe borderline sadistic, but I am not talking about sexual gratification. They did things for their own amusement. At least it seemed that way to us, the students. One evening we were practicing a kata (form) when our sensei told us it was wrong and asked us who had taught us to do it that way. Well, of course he had, but we could not say that. We all stood in silence. Soon he broke the silence and showed us a different way. Not skipping a heartbeat, we were expected to perform the kata from hence forward the new way. It did not matter that we had been doing it the old way for years. Later in the locker room, we all agreed that we had learned and remembered the kata correctly. We concluded we were being taught patience, to accept and change, and never question the teacher. During class I saw the "trap" set many times and witnessed many students fall prey to it. Those times when students fell for the trick, a smile came across my teacher's face. So I conclude, martial arts instructors are borderline sadists. And I am happy to pass that along.

In defense of disrupting the routines that my slave conjures up, I intentionally do so for her development as a person. The humorous side of sadism does not have to be just about the amusement of the sadist; slaves can learn to better themselves as human beings. Yeah, sure, it may take them some time to figure this out. You may even have to tell them you are teaching and testing them. Count on the slave forgetting this over time, though. Even after years of being with me, my slave still makes that same funny face whenever I strike that nerve.

My corruption is not limited to my own slave and friends. With permission, I will tease others. For me it is like flirting, a more mild form of sadistic foreplay. I was once invited to teach for a very structured organization. By this I mean they were very formal with strictly prescribed manners and etiquette. At a reception held in my honor, there were servers dressed in long-sleeve button-down white shirts, black pants, and bare feet. They went so far as to provide me with a personal attendant. As I stated before, I will scene with anybody when I have permission. That evening I asked for permission to mess with the servers and was granted such.

The servers were taught well. They came around with the different trays at regular intervals and each time, I said "No, thank you." We had just returned from eating Chinese food at a wonderful restaurant and I was actually very full already. But they kept coming by with the food, and I kept saying, "No, thank you." Thus, a pattern was established. So one server took it upon her own judgment to bypass me. Big mistake.

Naturally, I had to comment, "Oh, what? Now you aren't going to offer me anything?" She turned such a brilliant color of red. Stuttering for an explanation, I interrupted with, "You think because I said no every time before, I would continue to?" Fumbling for words, she noticed I had a big smile on my face.

"I am very sorry, Sir," she stated as she leaned forward to offer her tray to me.

"No, thank you."

Masters, slaves, and SM Sex

Inspired by Master Bert, slave nadine, and the 2006
South West Leather Conference

As I write this, I sit in an airport terminal in Chicago. Yet another delayed flight while trying to return home from the 2006 South West Leather Conference (SWLC). It was a long two days of spiritual endeavors. I was part of the piercing team for what was called the "Dance of Souls," a ritual full of drums, hooks, bells, and cheek piercings. After I completed my last piercing, I prepped my own flesh for hooks to be inserted. I gathered my supplies, entered the sacred space, and searched for a space of my own. I found it at the center of the energy where the drums were situated. It was there that I knelt down and placed my own eight-gauge hooks.

To put two eight-gauge hooks in myself was an interesting experience. It brought me back to the time I first cut myself. But with more knowledge this time, it was like topping myself. During other rites of passage, I had been able to separate myself from the sensation, but this time I could not. Part of me had to perform the piercing; thus part of me had to "be there." I felt sensation this time.

This ritual was not like the others for me. I did not "feel" much during the dance. Rather, it hit me while walking through the Chicago O'Hare airport surrounded by thousands of people.

Maybe this time, since I had opened my own flesh, it opened my own mind to new thoughts and ideas. Oh, heck with it – the why does not matter. The important thing is that I hope this chapter may enable others to utilize their relationships and sexual interactions as tools to assist them with leaving yesterday behind to live today.

The SWLC ended Sunday, but I hung around for another day to teach a class for the Arizona Power Exchange (APEX). The generous Master Bert and slave nadine opened their home to me on Sunday and Monday nights. We had a few opportunities to talk a little about Master/slave relations.

Master Bert told me he did not use sadism as a primary tool for personal growth in his slave; he has other methods. It was this conversation, combined with my self-piercing, that flooded my mind with theories while walking through the airport.

Because of my martial arts background which included some hard and fast teaching/learning techniques, I take this same approach with my slave and with teaching students. Traditional Japanese martial arts teaching methods can be very much like sadism without the sexual gratification. For example, if a child began to cry in class, we were to bring them to the front of the class for everyone to watch. This was very humiliating for the child, but it stopped the crying every time. There are circumstances when I will use humiliation, shame, and peer pressure as teaching tools in and out of a scene. I use these same techniques to teach nurses and paraprofessionals with amazing results.

I talk about "just being" in life, as well as using SM scenes for personal growth. Many of us fulfill the role of teacher in our Master/slave relationships. Then it dawned on me – how can we just be if there are issues that are never addressed? How can we be fully in the present if we have not settled the past? There is not one issue in my slave's past that I would not deal with in the present. On the other side, there are M/s and D/s relationships that never deal with personal growth of the slave or submissive.

I think we can only begin to live and just be once the past is left behind. I do not think avoiding it, hiding it, or attempting to forget it makes it go away. There will always be remaining triggers that can be pulled in the present.

Likewise, if we continue to be ashamed of our past, how can we be fully in the present? Perhaps this is yet another reason I use sadism to facilitate personal growth. It ties in so well with fears. Long have I believed that people fear the past. As well, the Master or dominant may fear causing more damage by addressing the slave's or submissive's history. It is the love they have that makes them most qualified to address the past. I firmly believe that the love shared between a Master and slave can overcome any abuse or fear. If the intent to help is genuine, then all will work out, I affirm. The present intent to help, love, and overcome will overshadow the past hatred. Believe in yourself and your partner and begin to live in the present, my friends.

When my slave came to live with me, I constantly hounded her to leave the past and continue as if it had not happened. After all, this is what I was taught to do. So why could she not do this? I have learned that not everyone can leave behind past abuse. We as adults can choose to let our past shape us into who we are today. I believe it comes down to a simple choice – listen to the past or not. But I also learned that some lack the "tools" to make and adhere to this choice. Why would a sadist even care about this?

I ascertained only recently the true feeling of what it is like (from my side) when a person gives in to pain and exhaustion. In the past I was able to sense when a person gave in to the control of another, but did not completely understand and absorb it. Again, this was at the SWLC in 2006. But it took profanity for this to finally resonate with me.

I was doing a long, drawn-out pressure points scene with a bottom, and during the aftercare phase, someone cracked a single-tail nearby. This triggered an emotional reaction and she literally took off running. Go figure — someone else had triggered a land mine. I tracked her down and calmed her a little. One thing led to another, and we were at it again. She was exhausted from pain and orgasms. Yet, I pushed further to take her up and down a roller coaster ride of pain and pleasure, and she was so wiped out she started to go to sleep on me whenever I stopped to let her rest. It felt right somehow, so I urged her a bit harder.

"Oh, fuck it," she said.

At this point, both the physical and emotional being were given to me. From then on, she was inhibited by nothing. There was no longer any land mine. She totally surrendered and that's a feeling that I as a sadist realized is a really cool thing because it is true emotion. There was no hiding. She finally surrendered her own will and followed mine. When people overcome their issues, their past and present worries, anything is possible. Then there's nothing stopping them.

Before, it felt like people gave in for themselves. I am sure I am wrong about that. But I did not feel it before. I place this responsi-bility on myself, however. I perhaps lacked the openness to feel the transition. So why do I say all this here? Allow me to bring it full circle.

My slave had issues with a past non-consensual rape at knife-point. I hoped that she would leave it behind her when I wished to do a knife scene or a consensual rape scene. But I knew if I went in that direction, something bad might surface. I did it anyway. I chose to truly walk on the edge. I would not let past issues inhibit the scene. We worked through it together, and now, while something I do to her may bring up a memory, the land mine has been defused, and we can have sex with knives, which increases her intensity level.

With all the intentional addressing of past issues in my scenes, not one partner has had ill effects. On the contrary, they have changed their lives for the better. No, this is not some ego trip I am on. I must attribute the "success rate" to the emotions, heart, and spirit that both my partners and I invest in one another. Love conquers all. Damn, how I hated that saying whenever I heard it. I can't believe that I wrote it after it popped into my head. There is truth in it, though. At least I can find one application.

Love conquers all … in SM sex.

Be sure you are not getting in over your head. Sometimes things come out that may require professional help – but you never know about those things until you step on the land mine and everything blows up.

This all ties into my philosophy of letting a scene go where it wants to go. How can we walk the path of spirituality and unin-hibited sex if it is riddled with land mines of the past? Thus we have the choices of not planting the mines in the first place, removing them before we begin, or defusing them as we go along. You may trigger things, but eventually it will be a memory, not a trigger to a bad reaction – like running out of the room while a top is trying to perform aftercare.

But I feel it is a mistake to step over the mines or avoid the minefield all together. If we never deal with the issues as we discover them, they will always be there. Sure we may be able to avoid them for our own peace of mind … only for the next person to discover and for our slaves to have to live with. Well, that's not the right thing to do, is it? It is the past issues created by another that can interfere with your sadism or relationships in general. Kinda sucks to have that handed over to you, eh? In all honesty, I would not want a bad experience with myself affecting another relationship.

As a Master, I feel obligated to deal with any and all issues involved in my relationship. This includes the unpleasant ones of the past as well. A Master's duty is to facilitate the growth of those in service to them – more so as a sadist. Now this will sound like I am totally spoiled, but I want to have the type of sex I want, whenever I want. I think I stomped my foot when I wrote that. Also, I can't help but think the slaves are saying, "Typical Master."

There have been times I have watched other scenes in a dungeon. One thing that always makes me (the sadist) quickly move on to watch another scene is to see the bottom wiggling their ass after the strike of a cane. Part of me feels this is false emotion, meaning not emerging from the person's core. It seems superficial, like makeup. Go deeper and the teasing vanishes. Yes, I know there are those of you who like that reaction, and I have no issues about that. It turns you on, but only makes me want to inflict more pain.

There is no concealment of past emotion when you deal with issues head on. The feelings are genuine because they come from deep within the soul. The rawness of these emotions is what the sadist seeks. What better way to reach inside a bottom and touch their soul than by confronting the past problems that they have locked away for years.

Holy shit, I think I just had an epiphany as I wrote that. Maybe this is another reason why I inflict pain, because of what it brings out in people. Pain, when pushed and endured long enough, brings to the surface the uninhibited, raw soul of human beings. When two people can experience this together, it is like meeting on another plane. It is like cumming the exact same moment your partner does, only infinitely stronger.

And once the heart and soul are exposed, they can then be dealt with in a constructive manner. It is here that "Master" takes over and personal growth begins.

Now that I have had an epiphany, I wish to expand on why I seek to feel raw human emotions by inflicting pain. I have SM encounters with many different people. I would be lying if I told you all these encounters never affected my Master/slave relationship. It is my hope that those issues are now behind my slave and me.

As mentioned before, an SM scene is sexual to me. The primal aspect of intense scenes brings out the "true" soul. Since we are individuals, what arises is special and idiosyncratic to each of us. Thus, each encounter is different with its own energy unlike any other. This is what I have tried to explain to my slave.

Ever have an intense passionate one-night stand with a person you just met? It is a very different feeling than "making love" to a spouse of ten years. Certainly you can have that same intensity with your spouse after ten years. But I am sure you can admit that some sexual encounters feel more "real" than others, more real because you dig deeper inside yourself – as opposed to, "Cum already, so I can go to sleep."

I think this is why some of us interact with so many others. The craving and thirst for true emotion grows each time we taste it. For me it has become not about the "sex" part of it per se, but about what is felt during those exchanges. It is what is felt that will make one orgasm five, six, or more times (males, that is) in one sexual encounter. No, I do not practice Tantra or anything like that.

It is the emotion that fuels my multiple orgasms. Mind you, these are emotions fostered by pain. Is it all making sense now? I don't feel there is anything unethical to this as it pertains to my Master/slave relationship. And most assuredly these sessions happen with my slave with regular frequency. She tends to be sore and fears me coming near her for the next few days, however. But this did not stop issues of jealousy, though.

As a side note, I can't help thinking that part of this is common between consensual and non-consensual sadists. It is the "true" fear, suffering, and terror the non-consensual victim exhibits that feeds the sadist. How is that for a scary realization ... commonality of the consensual sadistic Master with Jeffrey Dahmer – that is, before he killed his victims.

By now I hope that you have realized that I write the same way that I experience life. Which is to say that when something enters my mind or happens to me, I write about it then and there. Well, I just returned from watching a movie titled "Hostel." An interesting note is that I wrote what you have read in this chapter before I saw the movie, particularly the Jeffery Dahmer comparison above.

The film was about an adrenaline rush through cruelty, but had nothing to do with sadism. There was this club, "Elite Hunting," in which members could pay to torture and even kill another human being. There were guns, knives, gags, blowtorches, and an assortment of medical items in each torture suite. At one point a member is speaking to another assumed member about what it felt like to kill another person. (Now here is where my slave got concerned.) He asked the other man if he killed them quickly or slow and drawn out. He imagined it being drawn out so he could "feel it" more. The soon-to-be killer wanted to feel emotion from the person he was going to torture.

Yes, it was a fictional film, but based on "true events," though the screenplay was fiction. But I sense they did their homework for this movie. I saw parts of myself reflected somewhat, like when a member cuts the achilles tendons of a victim, lets him loose, and tells him he can get away. Well duh, not very far like that. It reminded me of a time when I tied my slave up, handed her a vibrator, and told her to masturbate. Oh, she was tied so the sweet spot that makes her orgasm was just barely out of reach.

It also struck me that among those raw emotions that I talked about earlier, like fear, panic, and terror, I left out happiness and peace. I wish to feel all true emotions from others. These include the feelings I get when they have reached orgasm, spiritual wellbeing, and even joy. Please don't think it is just about me hurting and scaring a person to get my dick off. Hell, I have spontaneous orgasms when my bottoms orgasm. It is that joy of what they are feeling that I open up to, which in turn gives me all kinds of warm fuzzies to make me cum.

I think because a consensual sadist is concerned about this part of human experience as well, it enables others to interact with us. It is why slaves do what they do for us. Yeah, there is all the pain and crying, but there is also all the love and happiness that comes through on the other side.

This is yet another train of thought that surfaced shortly after SWLC. APEX had added a wonderful loft to their dungeon space, which enabled spectators to watch scenes from above the main dungeon floor. This is a neat vantage point because it is less disturbing to those engaged in scenes below. As I stood and watched the various scenes, I noted to myself that many of the bottoms were having orgasms or at least appeared to be sexually aroused. Hell, the tops were doing their best to help them by using Hitachi Magic Wands™ and so forth.

There were some really nice scenes going on, some involving skilled and artistic flogging, and others with intricate bondage. It was obvious the tops put a large amount of energy into the sexual pleasuring of the bottoms, and took pride in their topping skills. And then it occurred to me last night (a week after SWLC ended) that I don't think the tops themselves had one orgasm among them – at least none that I could tell. Were they even becoming sexually aroused? I will add that there were both female and male tops and bottoms, so the entire spectrum of BDSM folks was covered.

This prompted me to think about my own scene in that very dungeon the same night. Yes, I was focused on my bottom having orgasms — it helped her be intermittently distracted from the pain — which caused me to orgasm more than once.

When it comes to consensual sadism, I think sadists are more concerned about their own orgasms than they are about the bottom's. Now why was I perhaps the only top to orgasm in the dungeon that night?

Dungeon rules can prevent a male in particular from having an orgasm in a public dungeon. My orgasms that night occurred while I was clothed from the waist down. For some males and females, the "necessary physical stimulation" required for them to orgasm, like masturbation and hand-to-genital contact, is not permitted. And, well, some people have problems with orgasms period. Hopefully some were at least sexually aroused.

Also, there may be issues of stage fright or performance anxiety. This is undoubtedly a psychological issue. And yes, orgasms are more mental than physical, which is why I placed necessary physical stimulation in quotes in the previous paragraph. We all have the ability to orgasm without physical stimulation, which is why I am able to orgasm with my clothes on – it is done by feeding upon the emotions in the scene.

Having an orgasm that is both physical and mental can leave a mess in your clothes. For some, this could be an embarrassing side effect, especially if you are a female who gushes with fluid when you cum. For males, there is a way around this issue: masturbate before you go to the dungeon. In sessions when I cum multiple times, the tank runs dry eventually, meaning my body does not make fluid as fast as I am expelling it. In time, no more fluid comes out.

Side note here: Once during a long sex session with my slave, I had an orgasm while she was sucking my cock. She raised her head and looked at me kind of funny.

"What is wrong?" I asked.

"Nothing came out," she pouted. She thought she had felt me orgasm, but was confused.

I just smiled and shook my head. *There is no fluid left to come out,* I thought, *but let her wonder.*

By emptying the tank before we scene, gentlemen, we can help prevent a big mess in our pants. Sure there may be a small mess, but to hell with it. I have long gotten over any issues of messing myself so I don't masturbate before my scenes. Ladies, this does not work for you as well because those of you who are "squirters" usually don't do so with every orgasm. At least that is my experience.

And as far as getting your clothes all dirty, that's why we have washing machines and dry cleaners. Your material possessions can always be replaced. What can't be replaced is being drenched in cum, sweat, and pheromones while feeling the primal energy from your bottom who knows you just came as a result of inflicting consensual yet undesired pain on them.

It also could have been that all these tops got themselves off once they got back to their homes and hotel rooms. Maybe they later fantasized about their scenes, which helped them to orgasm in private. It could be conceivable that they went home and had vanilla sex after topping in public. But why does any of this matter? Why even examine it?

For some people, it is self-identity and they wish to discover who they are and why they do what they do. This book is intended to help them and those who love them. Believe it or not, there are people out there who disagree with sadistic behavior. I am not the be-all-and-end-all of consensual sadism.

As time goes by, I see and observe fewer and fewer people who I think are sadists. It could be that I am defending myself and who I am from those unlike me. During this quest, I am helping others to look at what they do and why. Could it be that they are not who they thought they were?

How can people call themselves sadists if they never become sexually aroused during a scene when they flog another, or don't get off on it later? I should add that an orgasm is not required to be a sadist. One can be sexually aroused and never orgasm. Damn, that must really suck, though. I think my balls would explode eventually if I could not cum during or soon after my scenes. In those scenes meant for catharsis, but in which I am sexually attracted to the bottom, it can be difficult to keep the sadism switched off. You can bet the first chance I get for release, I take it; whether that be masturbation or fucking my slave, that emotional and, to a lesser degree, physical release is mandatory. This release, however, involves inflicting pain on my slave or recalling a prior sadistic encounter.

But what of the tops who beat bottoms and help them to orgasm, then go home to have vanilla sex? They did not orgasm or become sexually aroused in any way related to the scene. How could they call themselves sadists? Causing another to feel sensations that make them cum does not make you a sadist, even if those sensations are caused by a barbed-wire singletail. The same holds true if you tie a person up, fuck them, and you both orgasm; this is not sadism since there was no pain, either physical or emotional. If they liked being tied up and fucked, you were not being a sadist — they never suffered.

While gathering information for this book, I talked to many people and asked them what they get out of causing others pain. In one conversation with a friend we began to talk about how he participated in SM porn movies. He remarked how he "only had to do SM and did not have do any fucking." By fucking, he meant he did not have to have any type of sex. I was very perplexed by this statement, because SM *is* sex to me.

This is the typical behavior I find in many dungeons. The tops seem to be there for the pleasure of the bottoms, because it seems they are the only ones sexually aroused. What kind of fucked up world is that? Sex for the pleasure of one person – that is not sadism. Oops, rewind. It is sadism if the only one cumming is the sadist.

Far too often, all I see anymore is kinky sex in public dungeons. I hope this is not a reflection of what people do in private. If so, we have diluted sadism into nothing more than sex with a blindfold and fuzzy handcuffs.

The consensual sadist feeds on the emotional suffering of another to get off sexually. We have become so lost in pleasing others in our dungeons and making it insufferably safe that we have lost sight of what the SM part of BDSM is really about.

Sadism is raw, primal emotion that can only be found by pushing your partner beyond his or her perceived limits to a state of suffering. If you always scene in your bottom's comfort zone, you will never know what sadism is.

A Word About Safewords

This section is not intended for beginners, novices, or the less-skilled. I am heading into a very controversial topic. It's thinking out of the box, thinking about where a few tops and bottoms boldly go, exploring the outer limits of their own minds.

For those who may be unfamiliar with the term, safewords are signals used to indicate that a partner in a scene has reached a physical or emotional limit. A safeword may be an agreed-upon codeword such as "red" or "yellow" or even "safeword" itself. When verbal communication is not an option, it may be a gesture, such as a foot stomp, or the dropping of a bell or a hanky held in the bottom's hand. Bottoms safeword when they feel they can't tolerate continuing with a scene. Occasionally, a top will use a safeword, but more often the top will simply stop doing what they are doing when they don't wish to continue.

Some consider scening without safewords very edgy. I give bottoms a choice whether to have a safeword when they scene with me; often they choose not to have one.

When I say "edge," what comes to your thoughts? Fear? Exhilaration? Perhaps doubt that such things should ever be spoken of, much less performed. As a bottom, you may be thinking *Can I do this and survive to tell about it? Will it hurt too much? Will they know when to stop, know when enough is enough? Why do I get off on this stuff; I must be mental.* This internal negotiation must be resolved before we can participate in any type of edge scene. Once we accept that seeking what we desire may be painful, once we no longer tell ourselves, "It's too hard; it hurts too much," we set ourselves free to reach our goals. As BDSM folk we must first come to the reality that we do what we do because we want to. It feels right to us, and well ... damn it, it feels good – okay, maybe not "good" all the time, but it gives us something we crave.

Perhaps the most risky aspect of an edge scene is the mental element. In extreme "role-play" we try to create an alternate reality for our bottoms. Using all our skills of "mind control," we try to make them believe that they are being burned or attacked, for example. But are we creating a false reality, or does the scene become a reality in itself? The mind, in all its power and might, can make us believe things that we might not ordinarily believe. This is why I have issues with the word "play," and I do not like to use it to describe what I do.

Pushing personal limits is edgy in itself. For people who explore extreme scenes such as flesh hooks or long-term sensory deprivation, negotiating a spanking may seem rather mundane. On the other hand, for a person with Post Traumatic Stress Disorder (PTSD) who was abused by means of spanking, this could be an overwhelming scene. The intensity of interaction is relative to the personal experiences of the people in the scene.

There is a great deal to learn from the mind and the spiritual world. Holding onto the physical world, many never reach it. But the spiritual world is merely a separate consciousness; you can safely journey to and return from such a place. Just because you are out of touch with your physical body, does that mean it quits working? In fact, one can be "brain dead" and still have a heartbeat. The primitive functions of the brainstem that are not used for higher cerebral processes will continue to regulate the heartbeat, blood pressure, and respiration.

As we scene, we may discover new worlds out there that we may never be able to get to on our own because a safeword is called. I have seen baby steps taken towards reaching limits, and I have seen giant leaps, both with good and bad results.

When one gives up one's safeword, the question arises: "Is this still safe, sane, and consensual?" Some may have heard the term "consensual non-consensuality." I stress that this sort of scene is for very skilled, highly experienced people and then only when complete and unwavering trust in the relationship has been established. Note that a relationship can exist for only the duration of negotiation, the scene, and its aftercare. And I believe giving up a safeword does not deny the bottom the right to stop an unsafe scene.

It is my contention that many bottoms call safewords far too soon. Bottoms will stop a scene when their mind thinks it can't take any more. This decision may be based on the level of pain they are feeling, or it could stem from the emotional stress of humiliation, where there is no physical stimulation involved.

To provide an example of going beyond safewords, I will relate a short story. In one of my classes on sadism, I wished to demonstrate physical sadism through a flogging. Mind you, the floggers were made of nickel-plated chain and purple suede. I had a DJ at my disposal, so I asked him to cue up two songs, both by Nine Inch Nails: "Head Like a Hole" and "Closer."

The flogging began without any warm-up. The bottom was showered about the chest, abdomen and legs with sharp, stinging blows.

Tears smeared her makeup. "Cheesecake" whimpered out of her mouth as she dropped to the floor. The first song was not even finished. Never before had she safeworded in a public scene. I held her for a little while.

"I want to continue. You have more in you," I whispered in her ear. "Stand up, please."

She rose to her feet under her own power, and the flogging resumed. The mini-scene continued for one more song (so they told me). This time the scene stopped when I desired to stop it. But only after she had dropped to the floor again, and I had spit in her face multiple times, flogged her armpits, and let her feel how hard my cock was. In the midst of all the pain, I placed myself between her legs so she could feel my cock. Instantly, she wrapped her legs around me. Yep, while in severe pain with spit filling her eye sockets, she was still willing to let me between her legs and she responded sexually to me – all after calling her safe-word.

Informed Consent

For many years now, our community has been discussing the controversial practice of "consensual non-consensuality" (CNC). If there's ever a dull moment in a discussion group or an online list, this is one issue – along with safewords and extreme scenes – that is guaranteed to liven things up. While I respect the concept, I think it's time for a more positive and accurate term.

I recall reading that CNC was a very heated topic of discussion at the National Leather Association's fifth conference in October of 1990.

In a post-panel interview conducted by Ms. Carol Queen, the late Tony DeBlase, the panel's moderator, was quoted concerning CNC: "A bottom may set parameters and say, 'Now, given those parameters, don't pay any attention to what I say after this.' We've gotten so much into negotiations and safewords that there are people who can't even conceive playing without them. They confuse consensual non-consensuality play with entirely non-consensual play – which it isn't."

This term has become no less controversial since then. There are some who feel it is in direct violation of the seemingly universal BDSM guidelines: Safe, Sane, and Consensual (SSC). When the phrase "Risk-Aware Consensual Kink" (RACK) was coined, it seemed to open a little more tolerance for CNC, simply because people were more willing to admit that there is some risk to many of our practices. But I have a personal issue with grouping sadism and "kink" together. Sorry, but equating the word "kink" to sadism is like comparing a bunny-fur flogger and a barbed-wire flogger. We all use catch phases to simplify our conversations, often using our local group's shorthand. However, once we start to travel or speak outside of the leather community, we find that interpretations vary widely.

Those who practice CNC generally do not use safewords, causing a portion of the community to promptly condemn the practice. Many BDSM practitioners hold the opinion that a bottom should under no circumstances ever give up the right to use a safeword. Yet there is an opposing segment in the leather/fetish community that chooses not to use safewords for various reasons. Some are bottoms who feel they cannot go as far in a scene as they wish to if they have a safeword. Perhaps an even more motivating factor is fear of the unknown. Some get off on fear, and not everyone gets off on knowing exactly what is going to happen to them.

As the owner of a consensual slave, I shall speak from this point of view. My slave has made the choice not to use a safeword when we are scening, or at any other time in our relationship; though she did cry "Red!" when I instructed her to eat a frog leg. She wishes to place total control in my hands as to what types of scenes and training we engage in. Many would call this CNC. I disagree with this description of my M/s relationship, and disagree with its use for any creditable relationship within our community. I understand it is shorthand, but I feel it is too easily misunderstood and harshly judged.

To consent is: "To give assent ... to the proposal of another." Non-consensual would be to disagree with what is proposed by another under any and all circumstances. So by logical sequence, CNC in SM would be an agreement to *not* necessarily be in agreement with the actions that are forthcoming. Some consensual slaves and other bottoms receive a great deal of satisfaction through unconditionally submitting to the will of another. It is through the process of giving total control to another that they achieve deep submission, leading to spiritual well being. It takes great strength and overwhelming trust to place total control into the hands of a Master or top. This exchange of power should never be done thoughtlessly. It takes immense self-discipline, enormous character, and responsibility not to abuse such power, once it has been given.

However, I believe that an individual who has consented to not using a safeword has not given up their human right to stop an unsafe scene. In what was perhaps the most defining moment in my slave's training thus far, she realized that she had human limits and that I would always honor them. To calm the mind and listen to the heart in the depths of pain, agony, and fear is difficult.

One evening my slave was boasting to me how she gave me total control and did not use safewords. In the midst of the conversation, I jumped up, grabbed a handful of rope and quickly took her into the bathroom. I began to fill the bathtub with cold water while I placed her on her knees and tied her hands behind her back. Grabbing her by the back of her hair, I pulled her backwards over the side of the bathtub and began to pour water into her mouth. With her back arched, arms restrained, and no place to firmly plant her feet, she was helpless. Quickly she gagged and started to spit the water back out. Her face stricken with fear, she looked into my eyes in search of understanding, only to find hollowness.

I stopped pouring the water and asked her, "Do you want me to stop?"

She replied, "Yes, Master."

What she did not know was that I could see, hear, and feel that she was no longer my slave but a human being with the raw instinct to survive; she had reached a very primitive limit. I did not intend to go on even if she had said, "No, Master, please continue."

I believe giving up a safeword is a declaration: "I will place my trust in you to do the right thing and I agree to your actions as long as I feel you are looking out for our best interests and safety. I give you consent, and I expect you to be rational with your actions. I do not give up the human right to stop you, should you deviate from this. Nor should you ever attempt to take away my human right to object to your actions."

This consent is given to actions with which the bottom or slave is in agreement. It is acceptance of actions that the bottom may not like, but trusts the top or Master to perform in order to aid the bottom's development as a slave and a human being. When a slave says, "I have given up the right to choose, say no, or have limits," they are giving their consent to allow another to have control, to make those decisions and judgments for them.

The above paragraphs are intended to explain why I think CNC is inaccurate. It is my opinion that what this term signifies is nothing more than informed consent.

In the medical field, we do stuff to people that they would rather not have done. Folks have elective procedures performed all the time which they know will result in pain, discomfort, and suffering. Why? Because they feel the results will benefit them. Are there risks involved? Hell, yes, that's a given. But they are informed of the risks. However, you don't see the medical field using terms like "risk-aware consensual procedures," do you? Risks are recognized; after all, body parts are being poked, sliced open, and removed, resulting in trauma – just like BDSM scenes. But damn, this is sex. Why do I need to explain that I have "kinky" sex when I am a sadist? I think more people are "kinky," rather than sadistic, though. I do think all sex should be consensual and informed as to how it may take place. And yes, you can inform a sex partner that you are going to do things they won't like and will not tell them about beforehand.

Anytime one says "non-consensuality," a forest of red flags is instantaneously waving. Mention consensual rape scenes or even consensual kidnapping scenes and the flags continue blowing in the wind. Many miss the word "scene" which means to portray roles, simulate, or otherwise act out. One is suspending one's disbelief and consenting to a simulation of reality. I am sure that when anyone in the legal system hears "consensual nonconsensuality," the non-consensuality part is blinking frantically, like an un-serviced neon sign outside a twenty-dollar-a-night motel.

Our bottoms, and we, as sadists and edge participants, have a difficult enough time just explaining our choice of lifestyle without having this added erroneous phrase nailed to us. The amount of control exhibited by a Master or top should never supersede the relative safety of the people involved.

In my slave's collaring ceremony, I chose to do a multiple piercing scene. Midway through the scene, she became very light-headed and warned that she might fall, yet she did not ask or gesture for me to stop. I could have chosen to ignore her worries but instead decided to halt the scene and render first aid. She would have gladly continued to the point of passing out for her Master. It was by the exercise of good judgment and caution that a potentially serious medical situation and/or injury were avoided. After a successful response to treatment, we were able to complete the piercings and the collaring ceremony.

Please understand that informed consent applies not only to sex, but also to other less invasive circumstances, such as the mental training of slaves and submissives. As a training tool at one event, I placed a restriction upon my slave that she was not to refer to herself as "I." For example, she could not say, "May I get you anything, Master?" Rather, she had to say, "Would you like anything, Master?" It was very difficult for her to follow this rule, and she became quite frustrated with her frequent mistakes. She disliked this training, yet she endured it knowing that I was teaching her something. It became even more difficult for her as other event-goers learned what I was doing. Soon they were enjoying trying to catch her messing up. By the end of the weekend, she was up to 72 "screw-ups."

I had asked something of her that she would not have been willing or able to do for herself, something she did not particularly enjoy, but she complied with my wishes because she trusts me to guide both of us in our M/s relationship. Later, she realized that the point of the exercise was to encourage her to place herself second and focus on my desires first.

By the way, I never did anything about all her screw-ups. But knowing she was expecting something awful was a lot of fun for me.

Whenever I begin to talk about not using safewords or about performing edge scenes, I always seem to get the skydiving metaphor thrown back at me by someone: "Once you jump out of the plane, there is no turning back." I offer this reply as one who does skydive and who also honors the concept of the basic human right to stop an unsafe scene. I took my slave skydiving for her first time. She and I went through ground school together. She learned how to put her rig on and check to ensure that all safety precautions were in place.

Now, let's bring "edgy" into this scenario. Say we are up in the plane at 13,500 feet and I think I packed her rig correctly, but she notices that I didn't. As a Master, I give her the order to jump. What should she do? Obey the almighty Master and jump knowing that the safety measures will fail, killing her? She knows how I feel about her human rights – I demand that she protect herself above all, even if it means disobedience.

Informed consent leaves plenty of room for what we Masters and edge people believe in – yet it still leaves our bottoms and slaves with their basic human rights and responsibilities. Our training and our scenes can still push their limits, but their limits as well as ours must fall within the bounds of moral, non-abusive, ethical behavior.

Sex on the Edge

I chuckled to myself the first time I was publicly labeled an "edge player" when the Beat Me in St. Louis event posted "renowned edge player" next to my name. It is not something I think about very often. But when I was teaching at the 2006 South Plains Leather Fest (SPLF), it occurred to me how much a sadist must scene on the edge.

When we talk about walking the BDSM edge, there tend to be two common interpretations with a single goal. Some will define the edge as pushing the limits of the person involved, whereas others will say it involves risking potential death or harm. An example of pushing personal limits would be doing a needle scene with someone who has a fear of needles. Pushing the death and harm barrier would include activities like heavy breath control and fire scenes. I think the end result of either challenges the bottom or sadist in life itself.

In order to make a person suffer, I think the sadist *must* push the edge. If you always scene in the comfort zone where the bottom does not suffer, how could you ever be on the edge? This works best with the personal limits of the edge; however, a person may be very comfortable doing a scene with a loaded gun, which could get them killed. Pushing these limits often causes emotional distress. Undoubtedly, for me it is the reactions to distress that I key in on as a sadist.

While at SPLF I was asked why I do scenes that could result in causing harm to another. I had told a short story of how my slave received a burn, which is healed now, when she backed away from me around a tree after I laid fire on her during a full-impact fire flogging. Yes, when we venture into the more hazardous aspects of risky sex, there is the potential for harm. But is it any more dangerous than driving to an event itself? I do not know of one person who has died from burns sustained during sex. But I do know of a couple BDSM folk who have died in car accidents.

I can't help but think the person who asked that question asked because they thought it was wrong to engage in sex that may result in harm. And I am okay if that person does not do what I do. Where I draw the line is when that person tries to tell me what to do in my life. No, this is not some revolt against authority; it has to do with what I want to do in my bedroom and my dungeon. Should we not do anything in life that may result in harm?

My point is that life itself is dangerous. We will all die of something at some point. I do some pretty treacherous sports, which include ice climbing, skydiving, mountaineering, rock climbing, and open water diving – all of which can get me killed at any given time. I enjoy the challenge, the view, and pushing myself to obtain something difficult. My slave follows me for her own reasons, not the least of which is developing her own sense of strength in simply surviving our adventures.

We don't truly know life until we brave it head on. If we never confront ourselves and live out of our comfort zone, how will we ever know what is truly out there? It is human instinct to strive to fly faster, climb higher, or dive deeper. Living on the edge gives us life; it gives us breath and brings meaning to what it is like to be alive.

Do I want to get killed or kill another while having sex ... well no, I don't. Nor do I want to get whacked by a car while crossing the street. If I had to choose a way to go, it would be while doing something that challenged me and helped me grow, versus what I would call a meaningless death. In the end I accept the potential outcomes of my actions and decisions in life. Some are willing to risk more than others for the gains of knowledge, growth, and self-worth. Why should these challenges not extend into how we have sex?

Because what I do is consensual, my partners are aware of the consequences of what they do. They also are stepping up to the plate to live on their terms. They do not wish to sit idly by as life goes on, just as I don't.

Facing Fears

The Bene Gesserit Litany Against Fear

I must not fear.
Fear is the mind-killer.
Fear is the little-death that brings total obliteration.
I will face my fear.
I will permit it to pass over me and through me.
And when it has gone past I will turn the inner eye to see its path. Where the
fear has gone there will be nothing.
Only I will remain.

Frank Herbert – "Dune"

Fear is a very useful tool for the sadist. Almost everyone fears something, and for good reason. Certainly if you ran into a bear while walking in the woods, when it began to growl at you, you would have a reason to be scared. The thought of being eaten alive *should* scare people. That is what we call a rational fear.

However, not all fears are rational. Some fears fall into the category of phobias. There are also many levels of fear between being threatened by bears and freaking out when locked in a closet. So at what level is a sadist to intercede? Is it unethical or immoral to work with severe irrational phobias? Oh yes, sadists, including myself, do have ethical standards and morals. Yeah, they probably seem lower than those of most of the population, but we still have them.

Over the years, I have discovered many fears that people have. This is a partial list of the more interesting ones: their bellybutton has no end, worms, bugs, having their feet touched, needles, eating baby squid, hoods, gags, fisting, pain, childhood, falling. But what I find that people fear the most is looking at themselves.

Folks tell me I am scary to scene with. My reply is that people don't fear *me*; they fear seeing themselves for what they are or once were. They fear I will show them what they are on the inside.

This was a discovery of mine as I searched for different ways to create emotional pain. Through casual conversation, my partners would open up to me about what frightened them. Sometimes I would obtain information through other people, as in the case of Heather and her phobia of worms. One fall, my student and I were teaching in Winnipeg, Canada, where Heather lived. I was to teach my "Awakening the Sadist Within" class, which is a free-for-all where I can show and do just about anything in the name of sadism. My student knew she would be eating worms during this class and had related this information to Heather, who in turn confessed her phobia of worms. She then stated, "You can never tell FifthAngel, though." My student is a switch and can be a bit of a sadist herself. The very next time my student saw me, she confided Heather's fear to me. In my student's defense, I don't think she ever promised not to tell me.

I had to find worms for my class, so we kept our eyes open while we drove out to where we were climbing that day. While driving along the Trans-Canada Highway in Manitoba, we ran across signs advertising "Nitro Worms." Now, I had no clue what a Nitro Worm was, but I needed to find out. On our way back from climbing, we pulled into the bait shop parking lot. I walked into the shop, greeted the salesman, and asked, "What the heck is a Nitro Worm?"

He said, "Oh man, you just gotta' see them. They are bright-green colored." Lo and behold, these nightcrawler-sized earthworms were fluorescent green. The man went on to tell me that they feed them a green dye as they mature.

"So is it safe for humans to touch and stuff?" I asked.

He replied, "Oh yeah, no problem. What are you fishing for?"

"Um ... I am not really getting them for fishing."

"Oh, what do you plan to do with them?"

I looked at my student and said, "You can take it from here," as I headed for the door.

To say Heather had a phobia of worms is an understatement. She had issues just saying the word. If she came upon a worm when walking outside, her dominant had to pick her up and walk her around the poor thing. She had such a fear of worms that she could not even make meals that required noodles because they reminded her of worms. Being the ever-caring sadist, I obtained her dominant's permission to use her for my class the next day.

Dinner at her and her dominant's house was interesting that evening. Everyone learned of Heather's worm phobia, so throughout the evening, everybody teased her. If there was ever a lull in conversation, we started up again with worm talk. The talking served a purpose, though. No, it was more than sexually stimulating; it was desensitizing her. She was becoming more relaxed with the issue. During our worm conversations, I had set a goal that she would at least be able to look at the pretty green worms without running out of the room screaming. Heather agreed she would do her best.

So why would a person agree to let a sadist scene with a deep core issue like her phobias? She knows it will scare her. She knows that I could make her worst fears come true. Yes, if I chose to, I could tie her down and let the green worms crawl all over her. Hmmm ... they could even be put into her mouth. Even inside her vagina. Boy, she must trust me. So, why?

Because she knows that her fear is harmful to her and it affects her everyday way of life. She will face her fears at the hands of a sadist, knowing full well I am getting off seeing her in emotional turmoil.

The next day at my class, I had Heather sit beside me on a massage table. She had brought with her the Nitro Worms in their polystyrene container. I ensured Heather knew every move I was going to make before I made it. I explained what the worms would look like. She knew what was with the worms for living conditions. I went so far as to tell her all the worms might be at the bottom of the container when she opened it. While I told her what to expect, she was holding the white 6" x 6" container in her lap. At one point she screamed and told me, "I don't think I can do this." I scooted over closer to her. She scooted away from me. Eventually I talked her into holding the box once again. Placing my arm around her to comfort her, I prepped her for removal of the lid.

There was no doubt in my mind that I was the one who would have to remove the lid. There was a small yelp, fidgeting, and then an "Ewwww!" Our goal was met. I was very proud of her. I was very horny. But I wanted more. Time to renegotiate.

"I think it would be great if you would touch one."

"Oh, no," as she moved away.

Cheers from the crowd urged her on.

"See that really green one on top? Just touch it."

Again she calmed down as I told her what to expect. "It will feel slimy. It will move when you touch it. Do you think I need to help you?" I knew this was a very big step for Heather. After all, the day before she could barely say "worm," and now she was about to touch one.

I figured as I held her hand and moved it closer to the green slimy thing, she would pull against me. So I asked if I could pull harder when she did. She said, "Yeah." As I edged her hand closer, I had to forcefully extend her finger for her and in no time, she touched it. Another yelp and cheers from the crowd. Heather had faced her fears and came through unscathed. We were all very proud of her.

Now someday, with a little more work, her dominant will actually get a spaghetti dinner.

As you read through this book, I hope you will learn there are many benefits to knowing people like me, people who are sadists who use their sadism to help others grow. Worms seem like a very non-invasive phobia to deal with.

Some fears come from our own making. Heather never had a "bad experience" with worms; she just didn't like them and the reason is unknown. But what was known to me was my student's past history of intravenous heroin use, a fear she thought she left behind twenty-five years ago.

My student had been an I.V. drug user but had kicked the nasty habit "cold turkey" on her own. But stopping heroin never changed how she viewed herself. She hid her little secret from my slave and me; even her girlfriend of nine years did not know she had been drug-dependent once. It was about a year and a half after she had become my student before we learned her history. We were having dinner when the subject of drugs came up. Eventually I pulled the secret out of her as she sat and bawled her eyes out. "Why hide it from me, your teacher? Worse yet, you hid it from your girlfriend."

"I am afraid people won't like me anymore." She feared people judging her because of her past. I would remember this night and address it later.

It just so happened that the same class in which I exposed Heather to worms would be the class where I would flood my student with a re-enactment of shooting up heroin – in front of fifty people who knew nothing about her.

Some fears are best addressed by telling the bottom what you intend to do. Such was the case here. She knew a week beforehand that she would be telling my entire class that she used to be a drug user. Before this time, only four people knew she had used. Another reason my student said she didn't tell anyone is because she felt she was "over it" and it was not an issue. If it was not an issue and if she was over it, then she would have no problems in my class. But for the week before my class, she would periodically weep over the pending ordeal. She would also try to talk to me about it. These were signs that she feared her past and what others would think. She feared my showing her past to her and what she once was. There was no fear of *me*. I told her what I was going to do and when. She knew I would do what I said – no mindfuck here.

I always do what I say and if I say I will do something, it is because I have the skills and knowledge to do it. And I have the nerve, self-esteem, and aftercare skills to do it. I hate mindfucks. They can be very detrimental when dealing with real issues. Also, because they are mindfucks, they do not allow for personal growth. All they do is "fuck the mind" and do nothing to help it.

"Tell people what you used to be."

"I used to be an I.V. drug user," she forced out while sitting center stage in the classroom.

A room of fifty people went deathly silent. It must have blind-sided all of them. I am sure they all were wondering *What the hell does this have to do with anything?* I went on to explain how she feared what they would think of her. Here she was teaching the class before mine as a nationally known BDSM instructor. Her class was about fear. Before I would be through, some of her worst fears would be realized. They also learned that she hid it from those closest to her. If it was no big deal, why not tell others, just as one would tell what foods they like or dislike? I tell people about myself so they may get to know me better.

"What does everyone think of this?" I asked.

"Once an addict, always an addict," was blurted out.

A nightmare come true, in my student's eyes.

Should one stranger's opinion provide our vision of ourselves? If we listened to the thoughts of others with regard to our actions, you would not be reading this book and I would not be a practicing sadist. So let us dispense with the mindless opinions of those who don't count in our lives.

I knew my student's fears were surfacing. Her body language, trembling voice, and wide-eyed appearance were there for all to see as she sat before them. The tears began to run down her face as her lower lip quivered.

Placed before her were a needle, a syringe, a band-aid, 2 x 2 gauze, an alcohol prep pad, and sodium chloride for injection. She later told me she had thought to herself, "What is that for? I never used stuff like that." Sorry, but the medical side of me came out. I could not bring myself to let her use a spoon and a small torch. But I knew the re-enactment would be close enough. In the past she had used her belt as a tourniquet, just as she did in my class.

Being a student of human behavior, I found it interesting how her shaking halted once she began her ritual. She was getting her fix, which calmed her. I still wonder if others noticed the change as soon as she pulled her belt off. With the precision of an I.V. therapy nurse, she hit the vein instantly, pulled back for a blood return, and injected. The room silenced once again. Tears streamed down the faces of those watching – so much emotion in one room. How easy it would have been to flip my sadist switch.

My slave once asked me if I want to have sex with the person I am doing things to. No, not always. There is no sexual relationship between my student and me. I was not sexually attracted to her. She was my student, period. Could I have flipped the sadist switch and taken it out on another? In a heartbeat. This was emotional fear and pain provided by me. The only difference was this was my student and she was being taught a valuable lesson. But I was to learn an important one myself.

After it was all over, I sat in front of the class to talk a bit. "So, what do you all think of me for doing that?" The responses were not much varied as some dried their eyes. In short, they all felt she was a very strong person for doing what she had done. Not one person voiced a negative thought of her past or my actions. None of this surprised me. Contrary to what my student thought would happen, they all thought highly of her. Including Ms. "Once-An-Addict-Always-An-Addict."

When my student sat down with the other attendees, she was showered with hugs and comforting gestures by those surrounding her. When my class ended, there was a line of people wanting to speak with her. I am sure it was all to give her praise for her strength and courage. Nearing the worship level in the emails that continued when she got home, fans spoke of inspiration and life changes they were making because of her actions in my class.

Yep, *her* actions and courage in *my* class. Noting a bit of hostility in my writing yet? All that time and still true as I write – not one person noted what I did for her. Perhaps I am being selfish for wanting acknowledgement for helping my student. Is that why I did what I did? So others would see me help her? What I learned was that not one person attending the class commented that she would not have done what she did without someone to put her through it – someone who cared enough to teach her.

After the above thoughts ran through my little brain, I concluded that I wanted people to see how a sadist could help and teach others. I wanted them to see and comment about the teacher role in the ordeal – not that it was "FifthAngel" doing this potentially dangerous scene to a willing bottom. People need to realize the possibilities that sadistic encounters can have for everyone. They need to see it was not just about one person … the bottom/student.

Adamantly, my student professed to me she would not have done such a thing on her own. So her courage was in trusting me to know how to teach her. If she had not stuck a needle in her arm, I'm sure she thought I would have. So was her courage really fear of knowing the consequences of her inaction? Who knows? What I do know is that everyone missed the involvement of the teacher pushing her limits. At least they never told me about it.

I beg of you to never forget the varied intentions of the consensual sadist, top, or teacher. Often, there is more reason behind a scene than what may appear from the outside – not just the thrill of pushing the edge. For some of us, it is not just about the fear or pain; it is about learning in life and helping others.

Do I think everyone out there should be dealing with such fears? Not a chance in hell. I have to deal with such issues as needle phobias in my professional medical career. This gives me added knowledge and experience with panic attacks, irrational fears, and how to deal with them. But I know nothing that others could not learn for themselves.

So always remember to thank your sadist.

More Sadistic Techniques

This is the part of the book where I give you a few ideas on how to become more sadistic. If you are a bottom, stop reading now and go to the next chapter. By some chance, if you feel you are sadistic enough already, then this chapter may bore you. However, if you think you could use a little help with how to torment someone, then by all means read on, my friend.

Throughout this book there are numerous detailed accounts of various scenes and interactions I have had. It is my hope that you will have picked up pointers from my stories. If you have not, I will do my best to explain ways to help you with your mind set and demeanor.

During a class on gun scenes, I was using a volunteer from the workshop attendees. I had picked a young lady who had a very real fear of firearms – so much that she was shaking and sweating before she even got on stage with me. For this part of my demonstration, I was using my Glock 19, a 9mm handgun. This is a very durable weapon that can take a real pounding. I mean you can run it over, throw it off a building, toss it in a mud puddle, and it will still shoot without a problem.

My victim walked up on stage, nervous as hell, trembling in her shoes, as I drew my weapon and began to wave it around while talking. I can be very animated when talking, you know. Well, this waving of the gun did not make her any more comfortable while she stood next to me. I don't think it instilled confidence in the audience either.

Next I extended the weapon to her, motioning that she should take it from me. Reluctantly she put out her hands and as she opened them, I dropped the gun. I think I heard a few cuss words shouted and I know I saw people ducking. My bottom almost fainted, I think. So what technique of sadism did I use? Incompetence.

If we look like we don't know what we are doing with "dangerous toys," it makes people kind of skittish. Mind you, the weapon had no firing pin or actual bullets in it. But none of that mattered anyway. It did not matter even when everyone knew the weapon was useless. The same reaction took place no matter what.

So one way to push the confidence and trust buttons is to drop things, say "oops" a lot, and generally look like you have no idea what you are doing. Very simple, and something we all can do. Oh, dropping things and saying "oops" when your bottom is blindfolded gets you bonus points.

Depending on the bottom, I may elect to be very outspoken or totally calm. When dealing with my slave during scenes (sex), I tend to be very calm, focused, and methodical most times. In rare cases, I will become verbal, such as in the episode when she got her worst caning.

My slave "upset" me by bringing up something she was having an emotional issue about. At least I wanted her to think I was upset enough to "yell" at her. We ended up in the dungeon – my entire second floor master bedroom suite. When it comes to punishment, I almost never use physical punishment. Rather, I prefer to use neglect. This time, however, I chose a caning. Immediately, she got upset because this was out of the ordinary.

I don't like wimpy canes. You know, the whippy kind that are about the thickness of a finger. Instead, I use something with some size to it. I want to feel like I have a big tool in my hand. My tool of choice – a 1" x 24" hunk of rattan called an escrima stick. It is used in martial arts as a weapon.

The caning began with my slave bent over her cage. Because this was to be perceived as a punishment, there was absolutely no warm-up. In physical pain from the get-go, her emotional frustration soon started. I saw an opportunity to escalate the intensity of the punishment: I brought up every "irrational" emotional issue she had shared with me over the past few months. I taunted her verbally and caned her harder with each blow to her ass.

Not to my surprise, she started to stomp her feet and occasionally pound on the top of her cage with her fists. It's a good thing the cage was padded on top; she might have hurt her hands. What was more interesting was she started to almost yell back at me. Never before had I been so verbal with her while caning her at the same time. This left her very confused emotionally.

You should also know that she was in no way restrained. As the punishment continued, in the process of the physical and verbal onslaught, she stood her ground of her own free will. I was very proud of her at the time. But I was not going to let her know that. To her this was all reality; no sex, no love, just physical and emotional suffering.

What made this so intense for her was my talking and yelling. If the caning was under different circumstances, I don't think she would have responded the way she did. I told her why she was wrong with regard to her actions and statements that had precipitated this "punishment." Very different from my non-verbal focused demeanor of norm. It was all just enough to tilt her emotions into a frenzy. To keep with the punishment theme, I offered her no aftercare. I simply left her in the dungeon crying with a black and blue ass.

It took great restraint on my part not to fuck her while she was bent over the cage. Her ass was so hot in temperature; it would have been so erotic to feel that on my cock and legs as I fucked her. Not to mention that each time I slammed into her already swollen butt, it would hurt even more. I fought myself to get these images out of my mind and the smile off my face, none of which I allowed her to see or feel.

Let me enlighten you further. When I write, I place my thoughts onto regular paper using a ballpoint pen. My slave then types this into the computer, later to be published. She just read the above about three years after I had done that "scene." I had never told her my thoughts or true urges until now. My sadism can be made to last a very long time. I told her that one day she would know the purpose of the punishment. True to my word, she now knows (and is probably making that "Arrrgh, Master got me again!" face).

It occurred to me just now that even though I am attempting to teach others about sadism, not all of you are going to agree with what I have done or will do in the future. We all have different levels at which we interact. We all have different relationships.

How I do things to make myself and my slave happy may not be for you. And, well, some of you may be way out in left field compared to me. I don't judge those who are different from me, and I ask the same of you.

Just as I often get asked how or why I am the way I am, many ask what they can do to be mean to their loved ones. Ever wonder why police officers never take their sunglasses off when giving you a ticket? Mind you, I see this as I drive by; I have not gotten a ticket for some time now. It can be intimidating when you can't see the eyes of the person reprimanding you. Not to mention you have no idea what they are really looking at. It is a good technique to help you detach from your emotions.

Another way is to become something you are not. As in the previous story: I was someone I was normally not. You can take this a step further by putting on clothing, masks, or even costumes.

Over time, I have developed the ability to shield my emotions through my eyes, just as you can or will learn to. "The eyes are the windows to the soul." This is true for normal people, but not the experienced sadist. When you become so focused on a given task, all emotions can become void when another looks into your eyes. What emotions am I talking about? The emotions that make people think you care. First, let me say I care for my partners enough to hurt them. If I don't like you, we are not going to scene. Nor do I scene in true anger. I may do my best to make my partners think I am mad, angry, and even downright outraged. Again, that is a character I take on to accomplish my objective.

My partners know I care for them. Before almost every intense scene with my slave, I whisper, "I love you" in her ear. My aftercare has a lifetime warranty. Well, I offer aftercare for as long as I am alive. But during a scene, I can't have my bottoms all happy with orgasms if I am to be a sadist. To show that I care would be self-defeating.

As stated before, there are times when they are happy to be scening with me; it helps them process. For the most part, the idea is to get them to a point where they are unhappy and I appear not to care about it.

Certain tools in and of themselves breathe sadism. For example: chain floggers, rubber whips, paper cuts, a shinai, bullwhips, metal paddles, and stun guns. But the most important tool is your mind, of course. Knowing what gets to people is your biggest advantage. Case in point, my slave prides herself on providing service to me and pleasing me sexually.

One of my fun things to do is fuck the hell out of her in every position imaginable, then not cum. What is worse for her is to be sucking and jerking me off for thirty minutes straight and I don't cum. I don't think I have given her a complex yet. Meaning I don't think she thinks she is not "good enough." Other times I will cum right away or multiple times during a session. But the whole act of my not cumming bothers her. After all, is that not how men have sex? We cum, then roll over and go to sleep. Worse yet, we cum and then just lie on top and go to sleep. Yeah, I have done lots of those things just to mess with her head.

While I have attempted in this chapter to give you ideas on how to be meaner, with love, mind you, read and reread my stories and the stories of my slave and partners. You will undoubtedly pick up other techniques throughout this book. To simplify once more, do whatever they don't like. Just have the courage and conviction to do so.

The Other Side of Pain

Long have I known that there is a place beyond pain – a state of altered being that can be found by breaking through the limits of human consciousness. Having been there myself many times through the endurance of suffering, I was passed the torch that I now bear with honor and pride.

We all need catharsis — a cleansing of the heart and soul. Coupled with fear and/or challenge, BDSM activities can strengthen one's character. What better place to be when full of fear than in the arms of someone you trust and love? Within the BDSM community we develop extreme trust in our relationships. Where else besides the military, law enforcement, and firefighting, or maybe extreme sports, do you place your safety directly in the hands of another?

What we learn in BDSM scenes can affect all other areas of life. During a scene we may inadvertently have to deal with fears, childhood abuse, or Post-Traumatic Stress Disorders. Emotional catharsis is a possibility in what we do. Whether it is a sought-for goal or an unexpected reaction, the top needs to be willing to be there to support the bottom as they deal with whatever demons are raised.

What happens to the individual who conquers these fears during the scene? Are they better or worse off to have discovered their suppressed feelings or memories?

Breaking barriers and conquering fears are not without their pitfalls. Poor aftercare, insufficient time and level of commitment are all factors that can make or break a scene. I recall countless times falling asleep on the floor holding my slave after a breakthrough scene. One advantage of having a live-in slave is that we don't have to part after a scene. It would be very difficult to place a time frame on aftercare. More so when you never know when cathartic scenes will take place; they just happen. Life has a funny way of going where it wants to when you let it.

When we break barriers we are by no means "playing." What we use are tools, not "toys." These life experiences are very real to those involved, with real consequences and real emotions. This is one area where casual dabbling and experimentation should never be done. I agree with the age old saying, "Plan for the best; expect the worst." I plan for the worst in every scene, as should you. You never know what you will uncover. You must be willing to finish what you have begun.

But how does one go from being a sadist to what some would call a "spiritual guide"? It really is not that large a leap. I spoke about detachment from emotions earlier. Also, as a sadist I have some really compelling fantasies involving hooks, chains and needles. My skill set of inflicting pain expands well into ways of helping others experience physical flight, i.e., hook suspensions. My medical background includes extensive knowledge of anatomy, needle placement, and sterile technique. And we'll throw in my climbing skills to help with rigging and pulley systems to make a well-rounded "spiritual guide," at least from the technical standpoint.

When it came to career choices, all of my adult life has been spent helping others. I progressed to the medical field by first becoming a lifeguard. From there it was Emergency Medical Technical school and on to Paramedic school. Last was Nursing school, which is where I have completed my training. In nursing, I have always been in the emergency room or the critical care unit.

Both areas expose you to the sickest people in the hospital. I constantly learn from patients who are suffering how a single event can change lives in an instant. We all learn just how human we are when we face injury, illness, and death – just how fragile we can be.

I don't claim to know the meaning of life or what happens next, if anything. But I don't think that he who dies with the most toys wins. (No intentional pun related to BDSM there.) What I see is people searching for meaning in material possessions, the right job, or the right Master or slave. While these things may make one happy, they never teach one to look at oneself.

Teaching is something I enjoy very much and have spent years doing. Martial arts taught me to look at myself from many sides, including from the inside. It is a goal of every sensei that each student becomes a sensei. This means that we are all taught to become teachers. In the medical field we work under the premise of "see one, do one, teach one." With this in mind, I choose — or rather I was given — the ability to teach others about themselves through pain.

But this ideation is nothing new; it has been around for thousands of years in countless cultures. And rather than recounting history, please just trust me on this one.

When I first started being a sadist, my partners had no idea what to think of me, though. I was never rejected for my sadism. You should also know that I had no clue why people let me do the things I did. Now I have a better understanding.

So back to why I inflict pain on others for non-sexual reasons. I would like to break this up into two separate categories. In both, the pain is a means to reach a destination. It is the path that the bottom must walk. I pave the path and bring them to the metaphorical gate. It is they who must pass through the gate. Yes, I give them a pretty big shove.

First we have rites of passage. By this I mean hook suspensions, hook pulls, ball dances, and so forth. To obtain a state of euphoria, these folks will endure what they must. For some the pain really hurts, while for others there is never any pain. There is a segment of spiritual travelers like myself who are able to separate themselves and feel no "pain" while hooks and needles are being placed. However, we still feel sensation.

When I help others with rites of passage, it is my technical skills that perhaps help the most. My knowledge of placing needles and hooks, combined with my experience in the medical field, tends to relax those taking the journey. I would be foolish to think that my heart and intentions have nothing to do with it. But when it comes down to it, I have no control over where a person goes. Because I suspend somebody does not mean they will meet their god, have an out-of-body experience, or see a spirit animal. All I can do is place them in the air with the best technical knowledge, love, and care that I can.

Because I know what can happen when people let go of pain, I use it for rites of passage. For whatever reasons, I have been given the ability to do what I do and I feel obligated to share it.

The second category is catharsis through pain. Although suffering may be incidental to obtaining a state of being, it is also a requirement for some. This is where it differs from rites of passage. As I stated before, some can separate from perceived pain before it begins. For catharsis through pain, one must experience the pain first and then separate from it. The best example of this is the scene that Rich Dockter and I shared. The scene was about pain, period. He wanted to know what it would be like to have no choice to stop feeling pain. He wanted to suffer.

Catharsis through this type of pain is more closely related to sadism because it is pain that I want to cause. Rather than letting it excite me, though, I flip off the switch that connects my emotions to my cock. I simply tell myself not to get a hard-on. So I don't. Sure, at times random sexual thoughts will enter my mind during such scenes. But I stay focused on the potential outcome.

Again, this is an outcome I have no control over. I can make anyone feel pain, just as any sadist can, but after that, it is out of my control. The bottom must let go of the pain, the fear, and the terror that they may be feeling.

There is a major difference between pain endured for a rite of passage versus pain for catharsis when it comes to loved ones. During rites of passage the loved ones and family of the bottom often understand and watch what is taking place. Conversely, to watch your loved one endure hours of pain at the hands of another can be heartbreaking.

Caning, kicking, punching, and flogging are examples of ways I have inflicted pain for catharsis. It can appear very brutal and even violent to an outsider, at times resulting in the observing loved one having to leave. Yes, I consider a loved one an outsider to an extent, only because they are not there in the moment with the bottom and me. While we may not want the scene to end, their loved one does. But the scene is not about them. It is about looking inside at yourself. The scene is about one person and one person alone, the bottom. But again, don't lose sight that a teacher/ guide is involved.

Certainly I speak to the loved ones and involve them in aftercare. It is they who will be with the bottom long after my work is done. They will see the bruises and may have to tend to them. It is they, the loved ones, who will also see changes that the bottom will make in life. People come out the other side with new perspectives; you will get a chance to read firsthand accounts of this.

So what do I get out of all this? This is a question I used to ask myself. Is it a selfless act? No. I get a sense of helping from aiding with catharsis and rites of passage. It is the teacher side of me that comes out. Often I cry during or after such scenes and journeys. They are tears of joy and happiness because I know the path my partners are on. At times I feel them pass through the gate to the other side. It is a peaceful place and one I have difficulty returning from each time I go there.

So are there any other perks to doing such scenes? Well, when it comes to catharsis through pain, yes. Because these scenes often involve hands-on interaction without any tangible tool, it becomes more intimate. That is to say that it becomes more personal, more "touchy-feely."

The techniques that I use come directly from martial arts and shiatsu. Both are areas where energy flow and the use of Ki are paramount. To feel high levels of Ki flow throughout my body gives me my own sense of euphoria. When I am able to expend more energy, I cleanse myself in the process of inflicting cathartic pain on others. I will tell you the truth, though. In cathartic scenes, the more energy I put out and the harder I can hit, the better it is for me.

To put this into perspective, I will tell you a short story about my scene with Rich Dockter. At one point I was punching and kicking him in the abdominal area while he was standing unrestrained. As I began to impact him, he would stand his ground. Eventually, as I hit him harder, he would be propelled backward. What was fascinating to me was that each time he fell backward, he stepped back up to the line to take more. Such an energy exchange was taking place.

There is one last reason why I do such scenes. Knowledge. I learn from what people tell me and what they write. Just as you will, I hope. Each of them stays within my heart and in my memories. They become a part of me, part of the family. But unlike your biological family or your leather family, this family you must earn. You must take that step to look inside yourself. To separate from the pain, this is how you become part of this family. And just as only a surfer knows the feeling of riding the waves, only those who have followed the path of pain and suffering know what it feels like to go through the gate.

The View from the Bottom
Pain and Catharsis in the Big Scene
by Rich Dockter

Rich Dockter – a man with impeccable honor and integrity. I probably have learned the most from Rich, more than any other bottom I have worked with. Because he has scened rather heavily from both the top and bottom side, he has a vast amount of wisdom. In the Aftermath chapter, you will read more about how Rich helped me. It was his knowledge from being a top that kept me alive, so to speak, after our scene, a scene that happened years ago that still gets talked about today. Rich, like Travis Wilson, has a gift for words. Just as he gave me his heart and soul in our scene, he does so in his writing.

Rich had asked me to present at an event he produces called "Thunder in the Mountains." I was a bit nervous after learning who else had taught at Thunder. Here I was, the new kid on the block at the time, being asked to teach in the big time. Rich did a little research on me by reading my website, specifically the origin of my given name FifthAngel. He proposed the idea of a scene with me topping him.

"I'm not worthy, I'm not worthy," was my first thought.

Okay, not enough pressure with the new kid teaching at Thunder; let's toss him in the fire by having him do a public scene with the event producer. A little taken aback, I was. But I was drawn to his etiquette and manners. He was a gentleman who spoke what he felt and thought, an honest man who would hide nothing from me. But damn, who was I to scene with a person of his caliber? Thus the courtship began – nine months of frequent email exchanges would follow, along with a rare phone call. It was for all the reasons above that I agreed to a scene with Rich. Everything inside me told me it would work out just fine.

The scene was to be about pain and nothing else. There would be no sexual content to it, so I really had to flip off my sadism switch. It proved to be very difficult to do, though. As the energy flow increased, my desire to tease Rich sexually was exponential. When the scene became more primal, Rich's will to endure the pain dwindled. This fueled my need to push him further to his goal of life after pain. The scene for me was energy in its purest sense – felt by all yet seen by none. One of the points that really urged me on was when I would hit Rich in the stomach with a punch, knocking him back. He would shake it off and step up to get whacked again. When the punches became kicks, his will gave in. I sent one final kick to his abdomen with the intent that he should not get up; he understood and stayed down.

It was this non-verbal language that bonded us in the scene, and maybe for life. We understood what we were doing and that was all that mattered, so we thought.

The lessons I learned by doing a scene with Rich extended to every heavy scene I do now. At times, the essay you are about to read is required reading for some of my potential partners. I do this so that others gain an understanding that a scene is rarely only about two people. As much as Rich and I wanted to believe this would be a journey for us, we learned it would also be a journey for those closest to us and those we loved. Indeed, this was a life-changing scene for me. Due to the impact and power of this scene on others and myself, I felt it only appropriate to give you both sides of exchange so you may learn what went through our minds. Following Rich's thoughts will be mine.

Even as a boy I was fascinated with the dynamic of pain. I suppose because I had been raised as a Protestant and because much of my religious training had been steeped in the image of a real man's body nailed to a cross and then deliberately abandoned to the hopeless agony that only crucifixion can produce, my fascination with pain arose less as an offshoot of masochistic curiosity than as a simple question of whether I would have been able to withstand the rigors and terrors of real torture with the same grace as Christ.

This is not to admit that I ever presumed to the same spiritual grace as Christ, but rather that I recognized that if Christ had been physically manifested in a human body, then he must have possessed the same vulnerability to pain as my own body. I wondered if I could have stood up to the challenge not as a spiritual deity but as a simple man. Later, when I understood throughout history how many millions of ordinary people had been tortured beyond comprehension, I wondered how I would have measured up to each and every one of their ordeals. But because I was no fool and understood all too well the real dangers of dropping into Baghdad or some other foreign stronghold controlled by psychopathic sadists to test my mettle, I found the next best benign substitute: the safe, sane, and consensual (SSC) BDSM community in America.

Suffice it to say that I was a fast study and that I jumped in with both feet. In the years since entering the community, I've bottomed for some of the toughest and best sadist tops in the country, and I've endured some very hair-raising scenes to say the least. But even within the strictly regulated and politically correct arena of SSC, I somehow felt cheated. I knew that as long as I was able to use a stop word when the pain or the brutality became too much for me to handle, I remained in control of the ultimate progression of the administration of torture to my body. And although I almost never used stop words in real scenes, I always knew I had the ability to do so.

None of the excellent tops with whom I've played would dare disregard a stop word for fear that word would get out that they were "unsafe," making it difficult for them to get bottoms to play with them again. This is the purpose of SSC, and it continues to work very well in the BDSM community. And although I was very aware of the alternative of consensual non-consensuality – of acquiescing to scene play in which there *were* no stop words, I had never yet allowed myself to invest that level of trust in a true sadist top (except for my partner at the time, and for whatever reason, he never chose to take me into the extreme realms of pain beyond endurance).

As a result of having bottomed so often and so severely during these years, I eventually became tired of fighting the challenge of pain and of having my body bruised and welted. I began more and more to top, but I still held out hope for the fantasy scene in which I would have no stop word and would be made to see what happened inside my head when I reached the point where the pain was intolerable but I had no alternative but to endure even more. I tried to imagine what would happen if I was taken to the point where I would scream to stop – where I would truly mean it
– and I were forced to go still further. Would I pass out? Would I

break completely and beg and plead? Or would I, as I hoped and fantasized, enter into that zone of catharsis where I would look down peacefully and with amazing joy upon my writhing body and experience a great and benevolent compassion for my own suffering but feel none of it. This, I felt, was what death must be like.

During my years as director of the Thunder in the Mountains event, I have always personally selected each presenter. 2002 was no different. I had already contacted the several return presenters whose abilities, experience, and charisma in front of crowds had set them apart as leather celebrities and whose presence I always desired at Thunder. But this year I was looking to find someone new and different. Grey, a local player who had attended Black Rose, told me about a new presenter he had seen who called himself FifthAngel (a name drawn from the story of the Apocalypse). Grey said this man was someone I should consider. I called one of my veteran Thunder presenters and good friend Lolita Wolf in New York and asked her for a reference. She told me FifthAngel was ostensibly a het player who owned a female slave and was very intelligent and well informed about his subjects. He had presented at Black Rose on the subject of pressure points. Lolita also said he had spoken in depth about the subject of intractable pain and catharsis. When I heard this I decided that I had to send this guy an exploratory email and learn more about him.

To make a long story short, he and I hit it off, and I invited him to present at Thunder. One of the two demos I asked him to present involved pain and catharsis, and because I selected bottoms for the demos as well as the presenters, I told him I wanted to bottom for him in his demo scene where there would be no stop words and where he could take me as far into the realm of pain as he decided to, no matter what I said or how much I wanted to stop. The thought that I was actually going to do this scene scared the hell out of me, but I knew that if I did not do it now, I would never do it. I was simply getting too old to continue pushing my body this hard indefinitely, and if I wanted this experience under my belt, I had better do it now.

At his suggestion (*insistence* might be a better word) we agreed to negotiate online and on the phone over the next nine months before the event. There were a few hard limits I imposed. Probably the most important one was that there could be no impact play to my lower right leg or foot. I had suffered a long bout of cellulitis to that part of my body and I had no desire to exacerbate the tissue weakness in any way. The 24/7 pain of cellulitis was significant and often disabling, and because my leg was now almost healed, I had no desire to compromise the progress in any way. In order to best protect and support my leg, I asked that I be allowed to wear socks and boots at all times during the scene. A lesser but still important "limit" was that no analgesic balm be applied to my scrotum. When I was younger, I had actually liked this burning sensation, but as time passed, it had become an experience that took me right out of the scene – I'm not sure why. It wasn't that I couldn't stand it, but rather that it put me into a headspace that made me want to walk away. It was not the sort of pain that fit into my cathartic fantasy, and although I considered that maybe a type of pain I really hated *should* be the one I experienced to take me to catharsis, I decided against it.

FifthAngel and I discussed many topics from trust to sex to playing in general. Because I was used to playing only with other exclusively gay leathermen (and FifthAngel was not exclusively gay), I could not help but wonder what sort of physical rapport we would have during the scene. With most play partners for whom I bottomed, I experienced an almost guaranteed amount of spontaneously easy sexual touching and posturing, and their sexual equipment was frequently used as a weapon of dominance in the scene. Because of this usual gay male dynamic, I almost always bottomed wearing only boots. As FifthAngel and I discussed this subject he made it clear that he would prefer to limit the play only to the pain and to its hopefully cathartic results and leave the sexual part of the scene to my imagination.

At this point in our negotiation, I had never met him in the flesh and had seen only one picture of him that he had submitted for our Thunder website, but even in the picture his face was covered by a sort of executioner's mask, and I could not really tell what he looked like. Lolita had played with him, however, and had told me he was handsome and well built. As a gay leather-man that was enough for me! It was only too predictable that both my libido and my imagination would work overtime trying to find a way to talk him into some sort of sexual contact during our scene. A hot straight guy? And in a public scene? This was almost too good. But as I felt him out in our emails, and as I talked to him about sex in general, I got the idea that he didn't want our scene to turn toward the sexual side of play. Even though I asked him, I am not sure what his reasons were. I think because this was his first year as a presenter at Thunder and because he was publicly identified as a het man owning a female slave, he may not have wanted to open the Pandora's Box of man-on-man sex at such an event. Such activity could go off in too many directions. He said he had played with men in other scenes at other times, so he was not opposed to it, but I think in this instance he truly wanted us both to focus on the scene's goal: attainment of a cathartic experience, and to leave our dicks out of it.

My partner Spike was not particularly happy that I had once again decided to bottom in a heavy pain scene. I had worn myself out several times in the past in such scenes and had ended up bruised and battered more times than I could count. It was always Spike who was there to watch me struggle back through the healing process and who was there to help me out when my body turned against me with cellulitis and the effects of HIV. Although I worked out consistently, ran miles each day, and appeared in very good shape, I was, after all, 55 years old, and Spike worried about my health. Although he did not come right out and ask me to withdraw, I knew he wished I were not going to do this scene.

On the Friday that Thunder began, Spike and I arrived at the Holiday Inn early so that we could be available for last minute emergencies and urgent management directives. I also liked to have some time to meet the attendees as they arrived and have a chance to chat with them a bit. As Spike and I stood at the registration desk getting checked in, a couple I had never met before walked up to us, and the man said, "Hello, Rich. Hello Brian. It is nice to finally get to meet you." It is not uncommon at Thunder for me not to know many of the people who walk up to me. The fact that I meet so many people at Thunder and other events each year combined with a rapidly waning short term memory often leaves me tongue-tied when people walk up to me with a certain familiarity which I am at a loss to reciprocate. For a second I thought this was going to be one of those times, but there was just something about this person that I intuitively understood, even though I did not recognize him by his physical appearance. I let my heart and my intuition do my thinking for me, and suddenly I knew this was FifthAngel. I have since often wondered how I knew him, but there was just something in his eyes that seemed to bring all of our prior emails to the forefront of my mind, and I had no doubt to whom I was speaking. We all hugged like old friends, and we decided that we would go to the restaurant and share lunch.

As we talked, I watched him and listened attentively. I wanted to see if I could find something about him that would make the difficulty of our scene a little easier for me. I think I was searching for that sense of trust I generally find in the eyes of those men to whom I eventually become close in this world, and it was not long before I found it in him. As we talked I discovered that I was becoming very much at ease with him and that I would certainly be able to trust him with my body, my spirit, and my right leg.

Something also occurred at the table during lunch, something that I had neither sought nor expected. I found I was talking a lot with FifthAngel's slave and it was through her, I think, that I got an appreciation of who *he* really was. She talked about the scenes she had done with him, about her fears and her attempts to either overcome or endure them, and about their relationship in general. Had she been too insistent about his kindness or his care of her, I might not have believed her and suspected she was trying to convince me of something, but she was very sweet, honest, and forthright which gave great credence to her words. By the time the lunch ended I was feeling very right about the scene.

Because Thunder is so filled with activities and events, it is always difficult to spend much time with any particular person, especially a presenter. So after the lunch I did not have much of an opportunity to talk to FifthAngel again. I had agreed to attend his seminar portion of *our* presentation so that he could introduce me as his bottom in the demo portion of the presentation that had been scheduled in the dungeon that night immediately after the doors opened. At the seminar, he talked about his techniques and about pain in general. He also brought out some of the instruments he used in his scenes and demonstrated his prowess with them. At one point he handed me the sharp katana (samurai's long sword) he intended to use on me in the scene later on. I remember wondering if he was familiarizing me with it or if he was trying to unnerve me as a sadist often does to his "prey." It was very sharp and seemed hot to the touch.

He also announced that he had earlier told me that I would not be naked during the scene, and that I should wear a jock strap of some sort, but he now revealed that he had only been toying with me and I could come to the scene wearing only boots as I usually did. It occurred to me that I might have misled him somehow about being naked in a scene. I truly never cared if I were clothed or completely nude. The truth of it was that because I had always bottomed for other gay men it was always they who determined what I wore or did not wear. Gay men are notoriously sexual in our play and always like to have complete access to any and all parts of the bottom's body. As far as I was concerned (except for the boots to protect my leg and foot), I wanted to wear what my top wanted me to wear because I regarded my body as a sort of canvas upon which he would perform his art. With FifthAngel I would have been just as happy wearing a jock strap as not. It was simply a decision of his by which I would abide. When he announced that I would wear only boots, it truly changed nothing in my anticipation of the scene. It would simply mean that I would have one less thing to remember and plan for, and I did appreciate that fact.

As the time for the scene rapidly approached, I became increasingly nervous and apprehensive. I went through my usual psychological "song and dance," upbraiding myself for having agreed to do something this severe. I knew I would be caused great suffering and I continued to feel guilty knowing I was causing Spike to worry about me. I always became nervous before a scene, but the nervousness always stopped completely once the first blow against my skin was administered. That was one of the things I liked about pain, and subconsciously that was probably one of the main reasons I had always enjoyed bottoming in pain scenes. The pain took me out of the realm of the mundane. Pain became almost a living, breathing being within me, and once it began to consume me, everything else in my mind and my life fell away into darkness. The only thing alive and filling my consciousness was the pain. And although there is no other way to describe it than "it hurts like hell," I welcomed it and embraced it.

It was like heroin that way. People always say that heroin takes away the pain, but in my experience heroin was *like* pain – once the effects of it took over my body, everything else disappeared, and in those moments of complete engulfment, I was somehow relieved of having to live in the world of things and people. I was solitary, alive only within the pulsing sounds of my own spirit. It was a place where I did not have to justify anything I was or anything I did. It was a place where I could finally exhale and where I could be at peace within my own mind. I have always thought that God had purposely made it impossible for the human body to endure such experiences for long. They had to be experienced in moderation in order not to kill the physiological body that hosted them. Heroin would certainly end up killing the body of the user, and heavy pain bottoming would eventually end up injuring and even killing the body of the bottom who did not have the sense to quit as he/she aged.

And God did this because He knew that for many of us, such glimpses behind the shroud would be seen as so soothing and so beautiful that we would want to live there always if we were allowed. So He created the effects upon our bodies to be so damaging that we would be forced to either stop or choose to give up our bodies entirely. I had run my course with heroin two decades ago, and intuitively suspected that on this night I would run my course, as well, with terrible pain and the beautiful pleasure it brought me.

I remember walking upon the platform that night about fifteen minutes before the scene was to begin. I was not yet in bottom mode, still acting as director of the event and making sure that all aspects of the dungeon and play party would run correctly. I wanted to shed this identity of control and pull back into one where I had none. There were people starting to sit down in front of the stage and many more milling around waiting for the scene to begin. FifthAngel showed up and started to check out the space that had been set up for him. We chatted a bit, and he asked if I was nervous. I told him I was always nervous before a scene like this, and he smiled. It was at this moment I could feel myself begin to pull away.

Before pain scenes, many bottoms need to take some time either alone or with their top to get into "bottom headspace." For me, it just happened. It was more of a function of my nervousness and possibly a function of my reason for being there. I liked pulling away and going within myself. During these times I did not want to talk to anyone and did not want to be distracted. But because people always seemed to talk to me nevertheless, I had developed an almost robotic ability to answer, smile, and say the things I needed to say without actually letting the words have meaning within my mind – and certainly without letting the words have an effect upon me. The closer I got to the scene, the deeper inside I pulled.

As the scene began and I stripped down to my boots, I remember FifthAngel walking up behind me and starting to talk to me close to my ear. He spoke in low tones, and because I could not see his lips move and because of a combination of the din in the huge room and my purposely having shut off much of the outside stimulation to my mind, I did not hear much of what he said. He pulled around in front of me and looked at me as if he expected an answer or a reaction, and I felt at a loss to give him one. I had no idea what he had said to me. Regretfully, I pulled myself back and asked him to repeat himself. He looked both a little irritated and a little disappointed, and I understood that he had said something to me that he had wanted me to take into the scene. He repeated himself and said something to the effect that he would always be *with* me during the scene, and I would never be alone. I had always known that about him, and had I not believed it from the beginning, I would never have gone through with the scene at all. But I was glad to hear him say the words to me and I felt even surer of him then than I had before. I suddenly regretted that I had not heard him the first time because those are the sort of words that should need to be said only once. I immediately hoped that he did not feel I was starting to let him down.

That was always one of my greatest fears in every scene in which I bottomed – that I would not be good enough or tough enough for the top to finish his entire painting upon his canvas, and I was certainly nervous about that tonight.

He stood before me and asked me to touch his chest with my hands. As I did, I felt the tremendous warmth radiating out from him, and I smelled his sweat. The smell of his sweat (any man's sweat) has always acted as an aphrodisiac to my senses, and this was no exception. But I was going deep into spiritual bottom headspace, and I rebelled against the impulse. I immediately pulled my hands back off his chest just far enough so that my fingers were no longer touching his skin but close enough so that I could still feel the energy and the heat emanating from him. In every pain scene, unless instructed otherwise by the top, I always kept my eyes closed. The way I saw it, I had no reason to have them open because the simple purpose of the experience for me was to feel only the pain and to fly away with it. Sight only helped to keep me tethered to the physical reality of the room. My eyes were now closed, and unless I had to open them for a particular reason, they would remain closed for the duration of the scene. Because I could not see FifthAngel, the heat from his chest seemed even hotter than it probably was in reality, and I could tell when he stepped back and away from me; my fingertips went suddenly cold.

He asked me to raise my arms over my head and allow him to fasten the wrist restraints so that my arms would be stretched out high over my head. Once the restraints were fastened, I paid little attention to what he was doing with them. Suddenly I was pulled hard by one wrist so that I was standing on my tiptoes. Immediately the other arm was pulled up as well. He must have fastened the suspension ropes at that point because I found myself standing on the very tips of my boots. I was not hanging, for I could feel the weight of my body on my extended ankles, but I was certainly stretched out tight! Because of the AIDS drugs I take, I have experienced the effects of peripheral neuropathy for several years now, and as a result I am very sensitive to and aware of my extremities – both hands and feet.

As I began to experience tightness in my wrists, I suddenly remembered my promise to Spike to be aware of my body and to not let myself become injured. I opened my eyes quickly to check if Spike was watching in the audience. I saw him sitting in a chair in the first row in front of the stage. His arms were crossed in front of him, and beneath the usual stoicism of his expression, I could sense a definite undercurrent of worry. I closed my eyes again. I knew he was watching, and the thought both comforted and worried me. It was at this point that a tug of war began within me that would continue throughout the entire scene. Because I loved Spike completely and because he loved me, I began to question whether this body of mine was still all mine to do with as I pleased. Did I still have the right to risk this sort of injury to my body when Spike was just as invested in my health and well being as I was? Was I being selfish in pursuing my personal and very idiosyncratic pleasures at the risk to my physical body? Suddenly I felt the way I used to feel when I used heroin. Who, beside myself, was I letting down? But as I felt the first touches of FifthAngel's hands upon my chest, back, stomach, face, and thighs, I pushed the thoughts of health and loyalty toward the familiar darkness beckoning from the periphery of my consciousness, and I allowed myself to fall into welcome step behind them.

Whenever I look back on a scene, some of the time elements become jumbled. I remember FifthAngel touching my body in a benign sort of way with cold/hot steel and I remember feeling the sharpness of it. Because my eyes remained closed, I cannot say what it was that he used, but when he picked up a flogger, I recognized it immediately. He began to flog my back with the familiar warm-up – a sort of tickling at first followed by more and more intense blows intended to facilitate the release of endorphins.

When being flogged, I tend to tighten up and fight the pain. Many tops have chided me, advising, "Relax, Rich, and let it flow through you." But I have learned to trust the responses of my body and mind. My back muscles and chest muscles automatically begin a dance of resistance against the restraints; with each new blow and each new pang of pain, I struggle harder and harder against my bonds. Inside my head I love the feel of the inescapable restraint as I rage against it and accept the heat of agony that flashes through my body. I pull and writhe and growl like an animal. As the blows begin to fall harder, I smile inside as I feel the sweat start to move to the surface of my skin and as I hear the first animal sounds escape my lips. "Here we go," I think. "Here we go."

I remember starting to brace myself mentally against what I knew would be a terrible onslaught against the flesh of my back, and secretly I welcomed the torment that would follow. But after a very short time, FifthAngel suddenly stopped flogging me, and I heard him toss his flogger aside. I remember thinking, "Well, that was easy. I wonder what's up." I honestly believed that he would pick up a heavier flogger and take off again. But he surprised me. Instead of further flogging, I felt him approach me from the front, and I felt sharp points of steel in my armpits. It was a sharp pain I was not prepared for, and it caught me off guard. I felt him push harder with the steel, and as the pain increased significantly, I began to pull up with my arms to retreat from it. But the pain followed me as I ran and danced into the air. I pulled harder and harder with my arms as I felt myself rise from my toes off the floor. I'm not sure how long I hung suspended, held in place by the knife blades in my armpits, but as he backed them off from my flesh and I felt the pain begin to subside, I briefly opened my eyes.

My feet were at least a foot off the floor, and I seemed to be floating high above him. I am taller than FifthAngel, but it now seemed as if I were looking down on him from a much greater height than reality dictated. His body seemed to shine and glow with a light of its own. I felt no pain and seemed virtually weightless. I saw Spike watching intently, and I closed my eyes again. I did not want to be reminded that he hated to see me suffer. I relaxed my arms and floated back down to my tiptoes on the stage. I remember being surprised at how fast things seemed to have altered during that one episode of pain. FifthAngel probed my neck and chest with the sharp

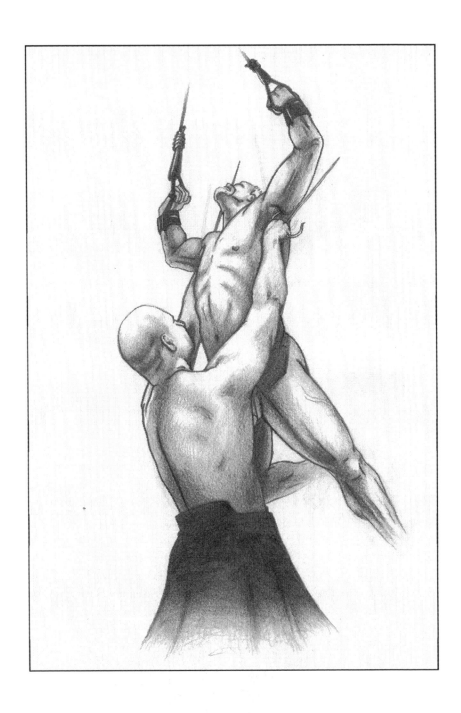

steel, but I could tell that he was moving on to something else. I was stretched out about as far upward as I could stretch, and I could feel my stomach muscles lengthening as I moved. There seemed to be a pause in the action and I could hear nothing from the crowd. My eyes remained closed. Out of nowhere I heard a loud "thwack" and suddenly felt a fiery pain in my left thigh.

Now, I knew he was using his bamboo shinai, and that the scene would begin in earnest. Another sharp pain in my left thigh – and then my right – and my stomach – my ass – my thighs again. I wanted to open my eyes so that I could see where the blows might land next and prepare for them, but how could I prepare for them? I kept my eyes closed and waited. The tempo increased along with my snarls and screams. I made no attempt to hold back my howls. The pain began to overtake my consciousness as I kicked out at my tormentor and pulled against the restraints holding my body taut and exposed. I could feel my mind begin to move within me and I could feel the familiar saturation that would override everything else. The pain was changing to agony, and I was reaching the point where I could no longer stand it. Subservience turned to anger turned to rage, and I felt the animal within me come to life. I pulled up with my wrists so that my feet were off the floor once again. The blows continued to rain on my body. I twisted and bucked as I prayed to God for respite, and amazingly it came.

For whatever reason, FifthAngel stopped his onslaught, and I hung limply from the overhead restraints. But now that the over-riding pain from the shinai was gone, I suddenly felt the overwhelming aching in my wrists. My hands felt somehow detached from my body – both cold and hot at the same time and aching horribly but at a distance. I opened my eyes to look at them and was startled to see that they had become blotched and purple. Maybe it was the fact that I was looking at them, but at that point, I suddenly knew I had to obtain some relief for that part of my body. My hands and feet were always problematic for me, and I simply did not want to take any chances of serious injury. I tried to stand up tall on my tiptoes to give my wrists some room and some slack from the leather that pressed against them, but I was stretched out too tightly to allow any movement. I whispered to FifthAngel that my wrists needed some relief. He seemed at once both startled and a little disappointed, but moved immediately to free my wrists from the restraints. I hoped he did not think I was using this as a ploy to escape more of the punishing work of the shinai. I knew I was quite prepared to go as far as he might take me, but only if my body did not give out and subject me to some sort of injury.

I wondered now what sort of restraint he might use on me for the remainder of the scene, and I was surprised when he asked me to simply stand on the stage facing the crowd with no restraint whatsoever. Secretly I was delighted because now I knew my will would be tested. I would have no restraints to pull and rage against, and while the idea unnerved me a bit, it also gave me the motivation I needed to set my jaw against whatever he had next in mind and attempt to hang in there and take it.

It was not long before I found out. He began striking my stomach with his hand. He was not using an open handed slap intended to cause a stinging pain. Instead, it was a hard blow intended to jar my insides and test the muscles that protected them. Over and over he used his trained expertise in the martial arts to break down my muscle tone. The harder he hit, the more determined I became that he would not beat me down. To prevent having the wind knocked out of me, I attempted to keep my stomach muscles tight at all times, but at various points in my breathing cycle, my muscles were more vulnerable, and FifthAngel seemed to know exactly when those points occurred. Each time he hit me, I staggered back a step or so, and then stepped back up to where I'd started and stood my ground.

At some point during this time I opened my eyes briefly, looking for Spike in the front row. I wanted to see his face and know that he was there watching. But my eyes did not find him. He was not where he had been sitting, and although I scanned the crowd in front of the stage, he was nowhere to be seen. I also noticed that a few other friends who had been sitting with Spike were no longer present. I felt abandoned and more than a little sad and worried. I wondered where they'd gone – why they'd left. But I did not have long to ponder these issues because FifthAngel quickly resumed his onslaught.

Before long he changed from using his hands to using his feet. Because he was an expert in such arts, his kick contained quite a wallop. With the first few kicks, he pulled his punch and tested me out. But as he continued to wear down my stomach muscles, his kicks became more and more forceful. With each blow, I would growl and groan loudly as I stepped back to maintain my balance. But as the kicks got harder, my legs became more and more unsteady. My stomach muscles were also wearing out, and each kick deprived me of more and more air. Finally, he unleashed the "mother of all kicks." As it landed against my stomach, I felt myself fly back across the stage. I remember falling hard against the floor, and for a period of time, everything went black. I felt like I was inside a barrel, sealed off against the world and deprived of air. I struggled to breathe, but no air would come. I struggled hard against the pain and at the same time welcomed the escape. Soon the air began to flow back into my lungs and the sounds of the auditorium returned to my ears. FifthAngel was kneeling beside me talking to me in low tones, but I had no idea what he was saying. I only knew I did not want to get back up for more.

It was almost as if he knew what I was thinking, for he told me to stay down on my back and to stretch out my arms and legs. He put new restraints on my wrists and on my ankles and attached them to the scaffolding surrounding the stage. Before long, I was once again stretched out, this time in spread-eagle position on the floor of the stage. Even with my eyes now open, I could only look into the blackness of the space above me. Now it was only my tormentor and I. I knew he would now push me into that space between life and death because that was where we both wanted me to go.

As I lay on the stage, I saw FifthAngel above me with the shinai once again in his hand. I felt a tremendous fire explode in my left thigh as the bamboo cracked against my flesh. Before I could fully comprehend the severity of the first explosion, there was another to the same area, and quickly, a third. I screamed and bucked in rebellion – this was too much. I wouldn't be able to stand the pain, but I had agreed in front of many witnesses that he was to continue with the torture until *he* decided to stop it. It did not matter what I said. Neither my choice nor my decision had any further role in the action. As this realization sunk into my brain, I began screaming out something I had never uttered before in a scene. I began to yell, "No, stop. Please, stop!" Always before, I knew that if I said these words in a scene in a way that showed I meant them, then the action would always end. I honestly think I uttered them on this night just to see if he would really continue or if he would give in and stop. To his credit, he acted as though he did not even hear the words and continued to beat me.

On one hand it was exhilarating to know that I was finally not in control any longer. I *was* going to be pushed as far as I could go, and neither of us had any idea where that was. As the blows continued to rain against my body, I remembered something that FifthAngel had said in his earlier seminar on this sort of pain. He had said that he was looking to take me to a point where he would be able to administer a type of pressure point pain that he absolutely knew would hurt beyond toleration and to which I would consciously register no indication of pain. In other words, he was going to fill me with pain until I was beyond feeling ... beyond pain. As he worked on me, I remember wishing that this point would come soon because the agony I was enduring was becoming unbearable.

I remember thinking that this is what had always set true torture apart from BDSM play: in torture the victim *had* no choice. I had always wondered if I could stand up to true torture as so many throughout history had done, and suddenly I knew that I could. It was not because I had any great capacity for endurance or for pain itself, nor was it because I was especially courageous or brave. I could stand up to torture as so many had before me simply because I had no choice. Once the choice was removed from the victim, he truly became the victim, and the only release from the pain of torture was death.

On this night I knew I would not die, but I did not know how far I would go before the effects of the beating I was receiving would convince my tormentor that he should stop. This scene had never been about *my* limits because without death as a final alternative and with no option to stop, limits are meaningless to the victim. The only limits that were being tested in this scene were the limits of the top to receive some signal from within his own psyche and from within his own spirit that would tell him to end the torment. And with FifthAngel I knew it would be when I would cease to indicate the signs of feeling physical pain. To him, that would mean that I had reached the point within me where my vulnerable soul, with its capacity to know pain, had fled my body and was watching the activity from high above the crowd.

As the blows continued, my mind swirled. Every type of emotion crowded into my brain at once. I was sad and happy. I raged against this man who tortured me; I hated him, but at the same time I adored him and loved him for having given me this gift of himself and of his spirit. I struggled and prayed to be free from the torment, but my prayers were also grounded in a sincere thanksgiving for having been allowed this glimpse beyond my mortal perspective. The alpha and the omega were both mine, and I embraced everything in between. I remember hearing the strange sound of water at the edges of my senses. As the pain began to consume me, I remember watching my body kick and thrash around mindlessly on the floor.

Then suddenly, I heard a snap, and a completely different sort of pain flashed a warning across my eyes. This was not the type of pain that I had sought to experience. This was a pain borne on the black wings of fear and danger, and in an instant my focus was ripped back to the stage and back to my physical body. A terrible and fiery agony shot up my right arm causing my shoulder to ache. I was *so* close to being where I had wanted to go and so close to knowing the answer to a question about myself that I had always wanted to answer. I tried to push the pain in my arm aside and pretend it did not exist. I opened my eyes and watched as FifthAngel brought down the shinai across my stomach, and the awful pain seemed to return with a vengeance. I screamed and bucked, pulled with my arms against the restraints that bound them. I heard a second pop in my arm, and this time I knew for certain that something significant had occurred, and it was not good.

I looked up at FifthAngel and whispered that there was something seriously wrong with my arm. His demeanor immediately changed from fierce and dangerous warrior to loyal friend and ally. Sometime during the scene, he had stripped down into some sort of loin wrap – something like a jock strap. I was sure it had a name in the martial arts manuals. He looked beautiful as he bent over me and ran his fingers down the inside of my arm, which we both could see was already swelling. I could tell from his face that he had made the decision to end the scene. He unfastened the restraints to each of my extremities, and held me motionless for a long time as I moved in and out of the world of happy delirium known only to those who have experienced it. He touched my body, paying special attention to my arm.

It seemed to take hours for me to begin moving in the world again. I remember that his slave came up to the stage and sat with us a while. We all talked softly, but I have no idea what we talked about. After a while, Spike came up on the stage, and I began to get dressed. I hugged FifthAngel and slave leslie, and we said our goodbyes. We did not discuss the scene much that night. I explained to him that I needed time for everything to find its place within my mind and spirit. He understood completely.

Later, I asked Spike why he had left during the scene. I asked where he and the others had gone. He confided that even though he knew I had wanted to participate in this sort of scene, it was not a scene that he could watch. My other friends felt the same way. They had not been able to see me hurt in this way. At one point they had even discussed finding a Dungeon Monitor to stop the scene, but knowing I would have objected, they simply left the area so that they did not have to watch. I understood that by following my heart and allowing myself to do this scene, I had somehow hurt Spike as well. It was as though I had kicked and abused his loyal and trusted dog, but in this case, I was the dog I kicked and abused. I had hurt Spike. While I knew he understood the dynamic of heavy BDSM play, I also knew that it diminished him to see me somehow diminished.

After two days of increasing pain to my arm, I went to the medical clinic for x-rays and an examination. The result of the tests indicated that I had torn the tendon in my right arm completely in two. It appears that I may have simply injured it the first time I felt the pain, and, had I stopped right then, I may have been able to save the tendon. But because I had made the decision to persevere with the scene, the entire tendon was destroyed. The doctors told me I could have surgery and have it repaired, but my arm would be in a cast for over six months, and the surgery was dangerous to nerves and vessels in the area. Complete recovery was not guaranteed. Instead, I chose to let the tendon heal as it existed and suffer only minor disability to the complete use of my right arm.

Upon hearing these results, Spike put his foot down and told me that my heavy bottoming days were finished. After thinking about the effect that this entire episode had on both of us, I decided to go along with him on this one, and I gave him my word. I had to come to terms with the knowledge that I would never truly know what it is like to be pushed beyond endurance into that enchanted land of catharsis and euphoria. A fascination I had indulged my entire life was now put to rest for good. On one hand, I feel like I have settled for less than I wanted, but on the other hand I feel that maybe I have come to terms with what it really means to be a mortal man. Not all questions have to be answered here, and sometimes we have to accept the fact that we get old and our bodies simply cannot follow our minds any longer into those lands where fools go and angels fear to tread. I am happy now with the choice I have made, and like so many other things in the lives of aging men, I leave it to those who are younger and stronger to answer the questions of life.

The Big Scene: Unexpected Lessons in Life

Shortly after Rich's email generously inviting me to present at Thunder in the Mountains 2002, he mentioned how much a statement of mine had intrigued him, a statement about pain. Explaining the origin of my scene name FifthAngel, I had written: "I was very much into inflicting intense pain – very slow pain drawn out over hours – pain that causes one to think of the pleasures of life ... or death."

We talked about the possibility of doing a scene together as part of my Spirituality and SM workshop. I was fascinated and honored by the possibility of doing a scene with the "director" at his own event, especially since he had never met me or even seen me in a scene. As any good bottom would, he checked my references, though I did not have many, and I checked his. I learned Rich was a heavy bottom who could take a great deal of pain. He had a national reputation built from scenes at Inferno with the likes of Bob Bender; there was something about fishing net and lots of clothespins.

Here I was, the new kid on the block as far as the "Public Scene" was concerned, virtually unknown to anyone outside Jacksonville, Florida. In my eyes I was a "nobody" about to negotiate with a major "somebody." *So why on earth does he want to scene with me?* Disregarding my inhibitions, we began the process of negotiation. He was in Colorado and I was in Florida so we exchanged information via email and thus began the nine-month-long process of getting to know one another. We started the usual way, identifying what each of us liked and didn't like.

In an email five months before the scene, Rich offered the following:

"As far as limits go, I don't have many limits or restrictions for tops to respect. I do not allow Deep Heat, BenGay, or other heavy analgesic balms to be applied to my scrotum. In earlier years, this was a big turn on for me, but for some reason it became a sort of sensation and pain that consistently took me out of the scene. The only thing I can think of when I allow this to be done is to end the scene and to get it washed off ASAP. And because of the effect it seems to have on me, I simply avoid it. This is a hard limit.

"I'm also not big on wooden paddles to my ass. This is not a hard limit and if a top chooses to do it, I will go along. I do like flogging, barehanded spanking, single tail, and especially caning to the ass. There is just something about the pain of paddling that affects me somewhat in the same way that the BenGay does to my balls – but just not so severely. If you want to paddle my ass, go for it! If you plan on breaking the skin on my back or thighs, I would simply ask that you respect the tattoos that exist there and try not to scar them too much."

Soon it turned into an intense search of his mind. I was combing the minefields of his psyche for information, looking for trapdoors that would inhibit our forward progress into the abyss. Meanwhile, being a sadist, I needed stuff that I could use to really screw with his head. He had sent me many photos of himself in various scenes, enduring what appeared to be very intense levels of pain. He was nearly naked in every one, wearing nothing but boots and socks. With the cunning of an experienced sadist, I decided I would order him to wear something over his cock!

His response: "As you know, I have bottomed in many scenes, but in all the times I have bottomed, I have never worn anything other than boots. I have always been completely naked. I guess that I have always considered nudity part of complete submission, and it occurs to me that no one has ever asked me to cover myself before."

While providing a complete medical history, he had informed me that he desired that his right lower leg be left alone. He had also mentioned that he leaves his boots on to further protect that leg. With my background in the medical field and shiatsu, I pushed the idea that I might want to work with his problem leg.

He replied: "I have never told anyone I would trust them to make the judgment about working on my lower right leg during a scene and making the determination for themselves on how to do it. I will give that trust to you, and for me, that is a big one. I want to go into this scene feeling one hundred percent good about you as a man. I want all hesitation on my part to be gone. I want to literally hand over all of my body for you to use as your canvas, and I want to know inside my most scared and frightened places that you will love me and take care of me. For once, I want to be able to go away in my mind and not have to maintain that very powerful and very subtle control over my own care and safety that all of us maintain in our deepest recesses. These talks help us to do that."

This kind of deep submission takes some bottoms further in a scene. To allow that which they would not "normally" allow to be done to them heightens their spirituality by deepening their service.

While negotiating this as a pain scene – Rich was normally very sexual in his scenes – I worried that he would not reach his maximum potential with me without someone cumming. I have a tendency to use my sexuality as a tool, yet not have "sex" during a scene. But we had agreed on a pain scene, so that's what it would be.

One thing that he had mentioned in his emails was that, even as the bottom, he was always in control. He could just say "no" to stop the scene. In the back of my mind I thought, *Yeah, right! If someone is tied up and they say "no" or they safeword, they are still dependent upon the honor of the top to stop.* It is the bottom's illusion to think they are in ultimate control simply by agreeing on a safe-word.

In an email three months before the scene, Rich wrote, "Because I top almost exclusively now, I find I really look forward to those special times where I consent to bottom to an especially good top. Even the anticipation becomes something of an adrenalin process where I experience the fear of the pain, knowing that I will reach that point inside myself where I will begin to fight it, where I will begin to rage against it, where I will begin to rage against the man who provides it for me, and where the only barrier in the world standing between me and the breakers at the bottom of the cliff is the exertion of my own will not to back away and stop the scene. You will find a man who wants to be taken down, however, and who wants to be humbled in a way that is very difficult to ascertain at first glance."

The first time Rich and I met physically was in the hotel lobby at Thunder in the Mountains. We had talked on the phone once just to say hello so I knew that he had a slightly raspy voice. He was a little hoarse – I was sure – from the past week of getting ready for his event. We were able to spend a little time together to get to know each other better in person. Lunch with his partner and my slave provided him with information on how I trained my slave. All the while he was hopefully gaining trust and reassurance that his decision for a "no safeword" scene was the right one. Also, we spent a little more time in each other's presence in my "Spirituality of Pain" class the next afternoon.

The dungeon was to open at 9:00 p.m. and the "big scene" was to begin shortly thereafter. I had arrived about ten minutes early to be sure that our space was properly prepared. At my request a special area had been set up – I was concerned about having enough room on all sides to wield my sword, shinai, and other martial arts weapons.

Surrounded by metal scaffolding towering nearly twenty feet above us was the stage where we would attempt to conjure up energy and achieve higher spiritual states. In preparing the temple, I had centered the restraints between the metal pillars to a beam just above comfortable arm's-length. After all, this was a pain scene; why the heck would I want him to be comfortable?

Preparing myself, I stood in the heart of the space where he would be standing, feeling myself in his place. The wonderful dungeon crew extended the stage to the front of the space to allow me full 360-degree access to Rich without fear of stepping off the two-and-a-half-foot drop. What a scene-ender that would be, having the top fall from the stage into the onlookers!

While I was setting up, people began to gather, moving chairs closer to the stage area. One very kind lady asked me if her chair was too close. Indeed it was, and I asked her politely to move it back. This became the anchor for a semi-circular seating arrangement in front of the temple.

To warm up mentally and physically I picked up two of my floggers and began to flog my image of Rich. Then with sword in hand, I ventured to the floor area just behind the stage. Performing a few kata and cutting exercises set my spirit into motion.

At last Rich had arrived and a bit of nervousness set in. For the last nine months we had been preparing for our upcoming time together. To prepare the audience, I had mentioned during our presentation that day what they would see at night. We had also mentioned in the program that this was to be a tough, heavy pain, no-stop-word scene. Sensing that preventing Rich from being naked would somehow impede his spirituality, sexuality, and submission, I rescinded my order earlier that day to keep him covered, and he removed all of his clothing but his socks and boots.

I sat him in seiza position in the center of our space and squatted down. The shining black leather of my hakama flowed around me onto the floor. I had put on my purple and black leather mask much as an executioner dons a hood to conceal his identity. Perhaps this signified my need to be detached, which would enable me to inflict the required sensations.

Probing into his mind, I requested, "Please close your eyes." Moving behind Rich, I wrapped my arms around him and pressed my chest to his back. Our first intimate touch felt very warm with the sweat already dripping from my body. Explaining my rules of no speaking and no touching without permission, he nodded his head in agreement. "What I do, I cannot do without love and caring. Never feel alone; I will always be here. Do you understand?" I asked Rich. He nodded yes, but only after I had to repeat myself, something I dislike doing. The noise in the dungeon had grown louder and, compounded by my whispering, his difficulty hearing me was understandable. Positioning myself in front of him, I too sat in seiza with his legs between mine. I closed my eyes and to my ears the dungeon grew silent.

"I will want to see you only through your heart and I will want to relate to you only through the trust we are developing as we continue our communication. And at the same time, I hope you will see me in that same light – as a human who happens to be a man and opens himself to you in a spirit of safe exploration and monumental joy," I remembered he had once written to me.

Lifting his hands to my chest I gave him a last opportunity to touch me during the scene. Shortly after contacting my chest, Rich moved his hands off me. *Strange,* I thought, *why would he not want to touch me?* Yet I still felt the presence of his hands upon my flesh. Opening my eyes, I saw that his hands were hovering just off my body. Basking in the forming energy, I could feel its intensity mounting. The stage had been set and we were preparing for the curtain to rise.

I sensed nervousness emitting from Rich and remembered him writing, "I am always afraid before a scene in which I know I am going to be hurt. Pain scares me, and I always fear I will be unable to give up to my top what I want to give him." Who could blame him? He was about to give up control to a sadist. I am not sure if people really grasp what it means to be a sadist. I enjoy seeing others suffer the pain that I create for them – I mean *really* enjoy it. This differs from the attitude of a Shaman; they understand the necessity of the pain they must inflict in order to evoke spiritual states, but they do not necessarily enjoy being the catalyst.

As I raised Rich to his feet, I realized he is much taller than I am, though I outweigh him by 25 pounds or so. While standing, it was easy for me to rest my head on his smooth-skinned chest. I secured his hands to the overhead chains with black leather wrist restraints. Due to his height, I needed to stand on a chair to do so. I dug my bare feet into the upholstered chair to prevent slipping, all the while thinking, *Okay, don't lose your balance and fall off the chair.*

With his arms stretched overhead and barely able to touch his boots to the floor, Rich looked extremely long and extremely naked. He had a pleasant smell to him, a natural odor, no perfume or lotion smell. I could see enormous veins bulging from every limb, humungous garden hoses that created a maze over his body. They were so plentiful they would make any intravenous therapy nurse drool, especially this critical care nurse about to top him.

Rich had superb muscle tone; it was not difficult to identify landmarks for acupoints. The thinness of his skin would prove to work well since it's difficult to press through thicker skin with my fingers. At times I have had to use additional tools to get to acupoints, but not with Rich. Each muscle was well defined; it was obvious that he took pride in his presentation.

When Rich moved from the various positions I had him in, I did not hear any creaking of his joints. His breathing was a bit rapid but not labored. I considered this consistent with the current conditions and his situation. After years of hunting and finding veins in literally hundreds if not thousands of patients, my fingers have become very sensitive to minute changes in a person's skin. Practitioners of the Asian healing arts rely heavily on palpation as a means of gathering information on a person's condition. I began the extensive task of compiling intelligence. Shivers ran all the way up and down my spine each time I felt one of those immense blood vessels.

During our email exchanges Rich mentioned that he did not enjoy his chest being hit. In examining him, I felt sensations from his chest that confirmed this warning. His upper back felt cold, as did his chest and the backs of his legs. His stomach was warm and so were his thighs. The light finger pressure I applied to those areas detected differences in temperature, emotion, and energy. On occasion I felt the need to kiss or lick a particular point, leaving a salty taste in my mouth. He had surprisingly tasty sweat. After completing my head to toe exploration, I concluded I would be focusing on his abdominal region and thighs.

Rich's abdominal area had a strong Ki, which told me a great deal about his personal character. He was a strong-minded and determined individual, yet kind and giving. This same type of Ki I have felt before emanating from switches throughout the leather community. One additional feature of his body was the wonderful artwork displayed upon it: primal tattoos indicative of meticulous attention to detail and the self-claiming of his own temple. I felt almost sacrilegious placing my own marks on top of this beautifully decorated canvas.

Time progressed and the pressure increased. The stripping away of layers to reach deeper levels of spirituality began, symbolized by the removal of my clothing. Peeling away the layers of my physical self, progressing ever outward to transcend this tangible realm.

During the day's spirituality workshop, I had introduced Rich to my sword, a Japanese katana. He had briefly become acquainted with its properties of gentleness and sharpness, but was unaware of its potency when combined with acupoints. Now, having felt his body and vital areas, I was ready to bring him into my world, the world of a martial artist and sadist.

I drew my sword from its scabbard. Its brightly polished finish always mesmerizes me and I'm drawn in by its beauty, its raw eroticism. With pinpoint accuracy, the three-foot blade repeatedly pricked his flesh, though no blood was drawn. As I touched parts of his body never before addressed in a scene, he was perhaps beginning to understand the potential of acupoints.

With a screwing motion I would imbed the tip of my sword into his groin, neck, and legs, slowly entwining skin with steel as I plunged deeper. I began to visualize the blade entering his body, the twisting motion opening the wound; I wished to create a reality in his mind of my vision, my fantasy. Jerking his head back, I drew the cold steel across his throat to symbolize a new beginning.

Deidoji Yuzan, a sixteenth century samurai, stated, "One who is a samurai must before all things keep constantly in mind the fact that he has to die. If he is always mindful of this, he will be able to live in accordance with the paths of loyalty and filial duty, will avoid myriads of evils and adversities, keep himself free of disease and calamity, and moreover enjoy a long life. He will also be a fine personality with many admirable qualities. For existence is impermanent as the dew of evening, and the hoarfrost of morning, and particularly uncertain is the life of the warrior."

Taking two floggers, I began to work on his back in an experiment. Was what I had intuited from his back true? Instantly his back arched. Shoot – I had barely begun! *So was what I had read from him true? Abandon this technique and go on,* I thought, as I removed my leather mask.

Stepping back to observe Rich, I felt it was time to use my sais. The sai is a trident-shaped steel weapon said to have originated in Okinawa. The center prong is about 14 inches long, while the two shorter side prongs, shaped like the horns of a bull, are about 5 inches long each. The three prongs can be sharpened to easily penetrate human flesh. In feudal Japan, legend has it that sais were originally used as hay hooks, but were fashioned into handheld weapons used to defend Okinawa from the swords of the ruling Samurai class.

I picked up my sais and quickly extended them, shoving the outside prongs into Rich's armpits. Immediately he jumped onto his boot tips, straining to pull up and away from the sharp points. I thrust further upward until his feet were completely off the ground. Lifting him above my head on my sais, I saw myself spreading the wings of a bird to the wind so it could fly. Rich seemed weightless, surprising me with the energy that we were accumulating. Guiding him back down to earth brought a smile to my face, though I doubt anyone could see.

A wicked little tool is the shinai. Used in the martial art of Kendo, or sword fighting, the ones I use are made from bamboo lashed together with white leather and measure 39 inches long from tip to tip. A gold string runs from the tip to the handle for a beautiful contrast in golden hues. Normally Kendo combatants wear full suits of flexible armor to protect themselves from pain and injury, though even through the thick protection they sustain some pretty good bruises.

The shinai I was about to use marks naked flesh with brilliant red streaks, though they would only be temporary and would not distort his tattoos. The streaks on the skin are due to the design of the weapon. With four pieces of bamboo strapped together to form a round shaft, it leaves ridges and valleys in its contour; thus when the tool strikes the body it leaves long red welts separated by skin-toned streaks.

Wielding my shinai, I began to work those fabulous thighs. I paced around him and assessed him from all angles, like a predator stalking its prey. While Rich kept his eyes closed, I randomly struck his ass, legs, arms, and stomach, an act of intentional confusion to prevent his mind from anticipating my attacks. I began with light taps, the ritualistic warm-up. At times it became difficult to contain my desire to let loose the fury of my weapon.

At last I felt he was prepared to experience the full potential of the instrument, though I still had to restrain my urges. I moved and knelt before him. I think he seized upon the pause in tempo to ready himself for what was to come. With a decibel level that could be heard throughout the massive dungeon, the bamboo slammed against his left outer thigh then again to the right with no time in between for him to react. I hesitated for a moment to allow Rich to collect himself.

Then another two deafening blows fell to his left leg with a pause to observe his feeble attempts to move out of my reach, to no avail. Another two blows were delivered to his right leg. A witness later remarked that the shinai could not be seen while in motion, but only when it stopped just a fraction of an inch from his body as it seemed to pause, then strike.

Having been in a kneeling position to deliver these strikes, I had made three perfectly spaced deep purple welts angled down each of his thighs. With the determined attitude of a caged animal seeking a way out, I resumed my pacing back and forth. The accompanying unsystematic blows to his body by the bamboo fell with greater force than before.

Rich spoke, "My wrist is really hurting," his words disrupting the karma of our scene. I released Rich from the restraints and allowed him to stand of his own free will. I saw this as a perfect opportunity to test his desire and determination to surrender control to me. Seizing the moment, I abandoned all my traditional tools: no sword, sai, or shinai, just us and the energy I would release into him.

I had long desired to free my emotion and pent-up passion through a punching scene. The intensity of such a scene can be incomparable. In this case, some called it "overt brutality" – the essence of human power demonstrated by two men through raw instinctive behavior. I had not planned for this with Rich; rather I flowed with it, as it felt right at this pivotal moment.

I began with very light openhanded strikes using the sides of my hands contacting him between his navel and lower rib cage. With each impact I felt him tighten his stomach muscles. He had his eyes closed and was unable to determine when contact was going to be made. At times I would intentionally wait for him to exhale and then deliver a blow.

We began to develop a rhythm as his stomach changed colors to a bright pink. He would inhale and tighten up, then receive impact and exhale. The cycle continued as the pace and force of blows increased. Gradually my power began to propel him backwards across the stage, only a step or two at first. By this time I was really sweating and the surges of energy were urging me further to catharsis.

All that surrounded us, the intensity of people watching, the energy of other scenes going on in the dungeon, all were being used. The tangible and intangible were incorporated into every strike to his abdomen. Drawing in with every breath, then releasing with exhalation and force into Rich, echoes could be felt by those watching. Of particular interest, each time I struck Rich and knocked him backwards, he returned to his original position in the center of the space. *What a connection we are making,* I thought as I stripped off my hakama. Now near naked myself, wearing only a cloth fundoshi, I was prepared to unleash "hell."

One witness stated he did not even see the next blow that hit Rich. As I am left-handed, I positioned myself to his left side. Reminiscent of the kata Tensho, which involves large sweeping arm movements, I struck with the palm of my hand, flailing Rich back five or six steps. Breathing very heavily, he slowly walked back to me and readied himself for another gut-wrenching blow. Again he took flight backwards, and yet again he returned. Again and again he returned for more.

The elements began to align for the final strike Rich would take standing up. I had used a few kicks already during the scene, delivered primarily using my instep. This technique results in a slapping, thuddy feeling. It was time to enter the next phase. Positioning myself in front of Rich, I inhaled slowly and deeply through my nose as I closed my eyes, absorbing all that surrounded me. Full of vital energy, I directed all channels to the blade of my left foot.

With the emotional and physical intent to bring him down to the earth, the impact of my foot to his stomach forced Rich back to the rear of the stage and onto his knees. Gasping for breath, he must have known he should not get up. I walked over to him, knelt beside him, and embraced him in my arms. *Does he know that this is only the end of this part, that I am only beginning?* I wondered.

Helping him to his feet, I returned him to the center of our temple once again. I laid him down on his back, spread-eagle with black leather restraints on all four extremities. I respected his need to keep his footwear on and was happy to place the ankle cuffs over his black-laced leather boots. I heard the leather creaking as I cinched the cuffs' buckles tight. Using the purple ropes I had prepared earlier, I secured the restraints to the surrounding metal scaffolding.

Now virtually helpless on the floor, the greatest shared sensations of our time together were about to be revealed. Once again, I reached for my shinai, the intended key to open the next gate. Still concentrating on his abdomen, punishing blows fell in quick succession. Each time he drew his knees up and each time they were met with the sting of the shinai, a lesson he soon understood. It was this part of the scene that Mr. Guy Baldwin would call the "agony" stage. Anyone who saw Rich struggling or heard him screaming would agree.

As I listened to his cries, I remembered an email in which Rich had offered, "I am not one to scream 'No, stop! Please stop!' if I do not mean it, and if I do scream it out, you can be assured that something is wrong and I do need to stop. Otherwise, I'll simply scream unintelligibly, writhe, buck, foam at the mouth, cuss, or do whatever else it is that I do to alleviate the pain within me."

Yet in the midst of the agony stage I stopped and peered down intently at Rich. Gently I placed both hands on my shinai and touched its tip on Rich's right wrist. He immediately ceased thrashing and lay still. *Unbelievable that we still have this unspoken connection!* Just moments ago, Rich probably would have gotten up and run out of the dungeon if he hadn't been tied down.

During the time he was restrained on the floor I traded off using the sais, shinai, and acupoints. I sat in seiza with his head between my knees. I put a little tension on each side of his head to let him feel that I did not want him to move from side to side. I inserted my thumbs into his mouth to access two acupoints. I wrapped my forefingers around the outside of his cheeks, which enabled me to constrict the points. Once again I inhaled deeply with my eyes closed and centered my upper body straight over his face.

With very rapid and intense focus I exhaled sharply, transmitting all the energy to my fingertips. Rich screamed in response, though it was not loud since his teeth were clutched tightly together. He became motionless as if paralyzed. My entire being relaxed, free from any stress or thought as I felt the same relaxation come from within Rich. I sat there for a moment holding his head between my legs, caressing his face. I leaned over and softly kissed his cheek.

I remember returning to using my shinai with the intensity still mounting. The spiritual connection continued until another disruption was felt. "Oh shit my arm!" He had unintentionally pulled very hard with his right arm. Immediately I removed his restraints. This distraction would not be overcome by simply releasing the cuffs; it was time for aftercare.

I do not know how long this next state lasted. However, Mr. Dave Rhodes stated that Rich and I lay in one another's arms on the floor for half an hour or more. Time was lost, as was place. With not a care in the world, I was unconcerned with anything around us, even in the middle of a noisy, crowded dungeon.

When we returned to reality, I placed the shinai in his hands while I held the tip. "Close your eyes and feel," I told him. He began to shake and uttered something religious. He and I were the only two to have ever touched the shinai since I bought it new specifically for this scene. The shinai was now his; he had earned it.

He spoke, "I'm sorry my body could not go on."

Upon arising from our drunken state, we were both grinning from ear to ear. I saw Rich looking over at my slave. She was sitting in seiza position, and apparently had been the entire time; her eyes were swollen and red from crying. I gestured for her to join us. Rich thanked her for her patience and poise during the weekend; she and I had not yet scened together. Kisses were exchanged and we embraced in a group hug.

Rich had asked me earlier in the day if we could put a time limit on the scene so that others could use the scaffolding for suspension. He offered 1 1/2 hours. I told him I didn't know how long our scene would last. After the scene, Rich remarked, "I see why you could not put a time limit on this." I just smiled.

As it turns out, those other pieces of scaffolding were never used. Not one couple scened in the stage area during our scene. I was told that at one point our audience encompassed almost the entire stage area.

The next day at my pressure point workshop, I asked why others did not scene in the stage area at the time. Typical responses were: "There was just too much energy up there." "It would have been an intrusion." "It felt like there was a physical wall."

Midori was the first come up on the stage and only after she had asked my slave if she felt it was okay to do so. Thank you for asking, Midori.

Though I am writing about this scene some eight months after it occurred, the vision is still vivid in my mind. The surges of energy still flow through me. Rich gave me a rare and precious gift and I can only be hopeful that I used it wisely. Rich and I both received emails commenting about how people's lives changed after witnessing our time together. My life was changed as well.

Another Remembered Piercing
by Travis Wilson

The first time I met Travis was when we were teaching together at an event about fourteen months before we did his hook suspension. I have to be honest here; he was overweight and could have stood to lose a few pounds. Nevertheless, he was well spoken and very experienced in the lifestyle. I respected him as a tribal elder. Travis is a very funny man and has no problem taking what he gives. What I like best about him is his "try anything once" attitude. I am sure he has fears, but never used them as an excuse not to do something with me. He is a dear friend and one of those folks I would trust with my life. He has even done a singletail scene with my slave.

Following are two recollections by Travis. The first is his view of a six-inch needle I placed through his face. This interaction was a large influence in my offering him a hook suspension. I think if he had not responded to the cheek spear so well, I would not have done the suspension.

The second essay is one that traveled the Internet at light speed. This was in part because of his reputation and credibility, coupled with the fact that Travis articulates himself so well it is no wonder it was featured in so many places.

So why offer an "old man" (his words) a swing from a tree using fish hooks? It was a year after we had done the facial piercing. During that time I had not had the opportunity to see Travis. When I saw him again at Camp Crucible, he astonished me. He had lost a great deal of weight and was looking fabulous. Before, having weighed what he did in relation to his height, I would not have done a suspension with him. But now, wow, he was a prime candidate. It was the combination of our prior interaction with his great new look that compelled me to offer. His great new look gave me a deeper vision inside him, which revealed his qualities of willpower, determination, and a desire to live well. Take it as a "Congratulations, want to hang from a tree?" There was no doubt in my mind that he would say yes.

From time to time the gods and goddesses decide to have a bit of fun at my expense. The first weekend in September of 2003 was such a time. I was at a lovely BDSM event in the beautiful hills of Pennsylvania, called Camp Crucible. This event is put on by Frazier of the Crucible dungeon in Washington, and is just a wonderful time, at the perfect time of the year – beautiful women, fun guys, gorgeous weather, tons of play equipment, more dungeons than I have ever seen, and an unending number of things to do. I arrive Thursday night and have a great time playing, teaching, relaxing, watching, eating, drinking, doing nothing, nothing, nothing that is strenuous or painful. Finally, it seems, I have matured, grown up, gotten wise, and set aside the foolishness of my silly youth, while I luxuriate in the process of allowing the young nubile women to serve my every need with me facing nothing more exerting than deciding what beverage to have next. Then comes Sunday afternoon. Sunday was the moment of great courage, spiritual growth, or overwhelming stupidity — you call it. Any of the above is right in my book.

A wonderful young man who goes by "FifthAngel" was another one of the presenters at Camp Crucible. He is outstanding in many areas, and one of his specialties is piercings. On Sunday afternoon he was doing an impromptu "piercing clinic" for just a few people. I sat and listened and watched. As he was finishing, he decided, at her request, to pierce the cheeks of his beautiful slave, Leslie. We all thought this was an outstanding idea, as it was "her" and not "us."

As FA pierced Leslie, my first thought was "Wow, I can do that." Some day I will mature to the point of not always following through on my "first thoughts." I asked her what she felt. (Yea, like in front of FifthAngel she would say, "Fuck this goddamned thing hurt like shit and I feel stupid as crap for trying it." Right.). She says, in this sweet little voice, "Oh, wonderful. It was wonderful. " You would think my own little voice would be going "Don't listen to that, Travis; she is his girl friend, his sub, his slave. She *has* to say that, even if they are on the way to the fucking emergency room, with her strapped down on life support." Nope, not me. Wise, elder of the community, Travis has to say, "Yea, I would love to try that. Can you do me next?" My son and every damn

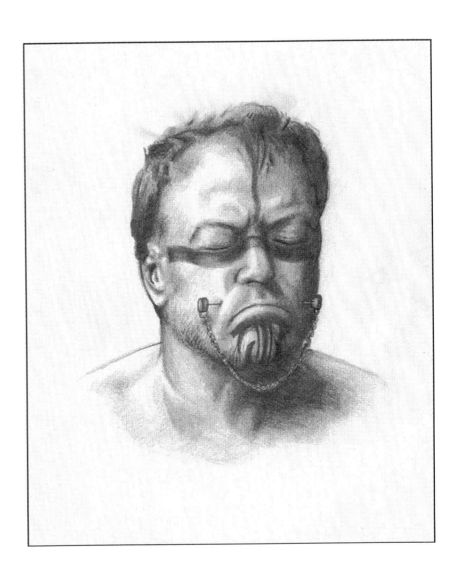

woman I have been with has told me I talk too much. Someday I will listen to them and shut my mouth.

FifthAngel, prick or nice guy, depending on your position relative to his needles, swords, or knives at any given moment, says, damn his hide, "Sure, glad to do it, come on over." Remember those words, and when any guy, needles in hand, says to you, "Sure, glad to do it, come on over," don't listen. Just go away. Far, far away.

I go over and sit down, and then, honest to God, something magic happens. FA pierced my cheeks. It was incredible. Never in BDSM have I ever felt an "endorphin rush." Never. I have tried. I tried with the Black Rose "Sundance style" chest piercing. I have tried in many ways. But never have I "felt it." I did here. And I felt it strong. From the moment the needle first pierced my left cheek, I was flying.

And it was not just a "nice" sensation. It was a "fierce" sensation. I wanted to fight. I wanted to go to war. I wanted to kill something, fight something. Someone looked at me and said I looked like I could eat glass. My response was that I ate glass for breakfast. Never in my life had I had that kind of "fierce, primal, warrior" feeling. It was simply awesome.

I kept the needle in for six or so hours. I loved it. I could continually get that same endorphin rush by merely twisting the needle in my cheeks. Over and over I did just that, and over and over, I went flying. I will do this again, many times. It will be a part of my "persona," a real part. This was truly a piercing to remember.

Kings Really Do Swing
by Travis Wilson

Once again, I opened my mouth to say one thing, and out came something else. But this time, thank you Lord, it turned out to be awesome. So awesome, that this story may be too "woo woo", or too "new age babble" for some folks, and if that is not your thing, this is a great story to pass up. This is all about "seeing a light," "communion with your gods," and feeling peace in an incredible state of nirvana. Yea, I am getting old. My mind is going, and my body went some time ago. But this is a story, a true one, that is, about an incredible experience that I had in the woods of Pennsylvania. I will tell you where it "felt" like I went. That is all I can do.

In late May of 2004 I went to Camp Crucible near Oxford, Pennsylvania. I went to teach some BDSM workshops and see old friends, and meet new ones. I had no idea at all that I was going to take one of the most intense and most joyful journeys of my life. Upon arriving at Camp, FifthAngel, one of the really outstanding Tops in our community, asked me if I wanted to do a back hook suspension. I was somewhat familiar with "hooks," as I had done a "Sundance style" hook pull at Black Rose some time ago.

That experience had been something special, but it never "moved" me. It was a "hill to climb," but it did not take me anyplace that I had never been. It may have been a "rite of passage," but not one filled with joy, or peace, or contentment. So, somewhat unsatisfied with what I had experienced on that "trip," and reasonably sure there was "more," maybe even "much more," I said, "Yes, let's do it."

I felt comfortable with this for several reasons. First, I trusted FifthAngel. I trusted his hand, and more, I trusted his heart. After this journey, I trust his spirit.

Secondly, he has taken his lovely Leslie on trips like this. She is the most beautiful, petite, sweet but intense young woman, and I felt that "if she could do it, I could do it." That is not an "if that little girl can do it, I can do it, too" sort of a comment. It is much more of an "I trust her, and if she thinks it is a good place to go, I can go there, too" comment.

Third, I was ok doing this because of some dear friends in Texas who took this same journey at various times in the past – Beth, George, and Leo. People that are dear to my heart, and people I trust totally. I thank them, as well as Leslie, because if they had not gone first, I could not even have gone second.

Finally, I felt ok with this because I needed to do it. This was to be the end of a Journey I have been on for some time. No, I am not stopping my entire Journey, and I will bore you with many more stories, but this was the culmination of a part of my Journey – a very special part, and a part that is totally private. I will not, dear reader, share the nature of this particular Journey with you, but I will say the following. By at least the age of forty, each of us has had their experiences in life that brought about great grief, great guilt, and great pain. Those experiences are different for each of us, and we each deal with them in one way or another. For some, it is talk with friends and family; for others, it is counseling, and for others it is some form of transcendent experience. It is that transcendent experience that I sought, and it was in Oxford, Pa. that I found it.

On Sunday afternoon, I met FifthAngel and several other folks that were to be there as supporters in this experience. Among them were Carla, who ended up being my support in more than a spiritual way; Carol, whose own spirituality seemed as touched by the experience as my own; and the lovely Barbara Nitke, the famous photographer, who took pictures of the event, and assured me that I did not look as old, fat, or silly as I might have. FifthAngel knows me, and decided it was a good idea to do a cheek piercing first. That piercing makes me feel awesome. Strong. Powerful. Like a tribal warrior. He and I both felt that if we did this first, it would assist me in dealing with the more traumatic back piercings – and his thought was correct.

He did that cheek piercing, and then I went into a bit of a meditative place. It is what I always do when "preparing" for something that I may have fear of. And believe me, I had fear of this. When I started the meditation, FifthAngel had me lie on my stomach to get ready for the piercings, and my fear was flying. I needed something to stop the fear, something to calm my body and my soul, and the meditation was simply not cutting it in the beginning. And then that cheek piercing took over. I began to feel like that tribal warrior. I got into that place of "fierceness" that this piercing takes me to. It allowed me to know that pain was coming, but that receiving it with pride mattered. And that thought calmed me and became my mantra.

FA (ok, I am tired of typing FifthAngel) then began the actual piercings: six 8-gauge hooks placed in a horizontal row across my upper back. No one ever did something with more gentleness, or more care, or more concern. But, gentleness, care, and concern aside, let me tell you something. Each one of those fucking god-damn hooks hurt like I had feared they would hurt. None of them was easy. None of them was dulled by the sensation of the previous one. They each hurt with a fire that burned all the way through my body, and if I never feel such pain again, that will be just swell with me.

But, and this is where it gets new age corny, once that last hook was in, that was the end of the pain. Nothing from that moment on was the slightest bit painful. It was not "pain that took me someplace," it was simply no pain at all. From that moment on there was joy, exhilaration, peace, intensity, but no pain. None.

After the last hook, FA had me stand, and wanted to help me walk to the "hoist" that would get me in the air. The last thing in the world I felt like was having someone help me walk. I told him I would walk alone. His concern was that I might be woozy from the piercings. I was not woozy; I was more in command of me than I had ever been. I did not need help walking; I was getting ready to fly.

He then attached me to the hoist and began the process of slowly lifting me off the ground. This was a "vertical suspension," so I started with my feet on the ground. (Ok, not my feet, my cowboy boots. Leslie talked me into wearing my jeans and cowboy boots as I did this. She thought it looked sexy, and when women like Leslie think something I do is sexy, I by God do it.) FA was trying his best to get me off the ground, but it was not happening, and maybe it was those damn boots, because what happened was I just simply kept losing my balance and fought to retain it. Maybe the cowboy boots kept me from getting traction; I don't know. I just know it was not working.

So I called to FA and told him I was not in pain, but I needed help with balance. He had Carla come over, and I placed my hands on her shoulders, and then he lifted, and it was so simple. I came off the ground, let go of her shoulders, and the second, and I mean the very second that I let go of her shoulders and was suspended off the ground, my world changed.

You have heard many stories of states of nirvana, of bright lights, of flying. Let me try and tell you not only where I felt I went, but what it felt like going there. What I am going to say is not, I suspect, literal truth, but it is the truth of what I felt. I will accept any scientific explanation you want to give me. I am not trying to convince you that what I felt was true, but I am telling you that the "feeling" was true, and more, felt like "the truth," as much as any "truth" I have ever known.

What happened instantly was the most beautiful bright light I had ever seen. It took over my world, totally. When FA had pierced my cheek in the past, I felt like a tribal warrior; now I felt like a tribal king, and I felt like a king ascending to heaven to be in communion with his God. I felt like I was in the presence of my God, and of others that I needed to feel (there was no "seeing" here, just feeling) and with whom I needed to share moments of silence and acceptance.

There was no sound, no talking, no messages (ok, maybe one, and that was again a feeling not a verbal thing, and it has been passed on to the one I felt it was intended for). But there was joy. There was peace. There was no pain, but a magnificent state of contentment. Ruined, I tell you almost ruined, as FA came over to gently swing me. I know he meant it as a way of enhancing my experience, because, yes it felt nice, but it also felt a bit foolish. Remember, silly as it sounds, what I was experiencing was the feeling of being that Tribal King – a feeling of almost total power, a feeling of incredible strength. And swinging did not feel very kinglike, I tell you, not kinglike at all. So I motioned for FA to come to me, and said to him, best I could with my cheeks pierced, hanging from that tree, that "kings do not swing."

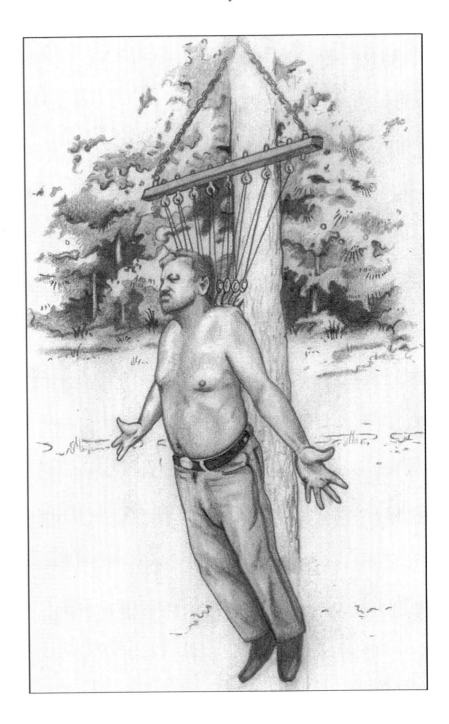

He understood and slowed me and then held me until I was still. And then one of the pivotal moments of the experience happened. Every single person that was there felt this. You see, the day had been totally calm – no wind, none at all. It was a lovely, cool day, but no wind. But within fifteen seconds of FA stopping me, the most incredible wind came up. It was not strong, but beautiful – cool, exhilarating, refreshing, and just enough to gently swing me.

I wanted so much to smile. I wanted so much to laugh. I tried to tell Barbara Nitke, the photographer, this as I wanted her to know the joy I was experiencing, as I was afraid that I might look in pain. But that damn cheek piercing would not let me say it without sounding like Mike Tyson after a Holyfield fight.

Why I wanted to smile and laugh was that what I was experiencing with that wind was the feeling that God, or the Force, or Mother Earth, or whatever you choose to call your own personal Power, was saying, "Yes Travis, for right now, you may be a king, but remember, I am driving this bus."

For however long I was suspended, I was alternatively "up there" and then would come back. When I came back, I touched those that were around. I held hands; I touched shoulders; I was hugged by several. Sometimes I would look around and people were crying, but each assured me that it was because they felt the joy, and they were moved to a beautiful state of joy as well. When I was "up there," wherever "up there" was, I was simply content. I could have stayed forever.

FA asked me if I was ready to come down. I answered that anytime was fine. He then told me that coming down was the hard part. Boy, did I misunderstand that. I suddenly was a bit afraid as he started to lower me, expecting pain. There was none. So I thought he meant that taking the hooks out would be painful. Wrong again – no pain there at all.

What he meant, of course, was that "coming down" from the experience would be the hard part, and yes, he was right. For two days, I basically wanted to be left alone – not because I was mad, or hated people, or was sad in any way. I was just in a state of peace that I wanted to experience, and did not want to let go.

Gradually that state of "peace" returned to a state of normalcy. I finished Camp (and it was a wonderful Camp). I spent some lovely days in Washington D.C. and had a lovely drive back to Houston. There were so many great experiences on a great trip, but among those moments that I shall remember for the rest of my life, was that experience of being a king, hanging from a tree, in Oxford, Pa.

Inexorable, Continuous, Synchronistic
by Hook

Hook (the name he took after spending some quality time with me) was my point of contact for the folks in Hawaii when I was headed out there to teach. We had talked a few times on the phone in preparation for my class. Occasionally our talks would drift away from my needs and into a more personal nature. To the point – Hook's personal concerns. He was very new to the BDSM scene and really had not found an identity. I explained the different positions such as top, bottom, switch, and that these were positions related to SM activities, but reiterated that they had nothing to do with dominance, master, slave, or submission, necessarily. He was somewhat relieved, I think, to know that I felt spiritual journeys like hook pulls were not acts of submission or servitude to another.

Hook was full of fear. He feared illness, being cut open, and most of all he feared the unknown. Eventually he asked me for help. Keeping him pretty much in the dark (unknown), I expressed that he and I would do something together, but never gave any great details. Why did I choose to help Hook? On one level it was kind of fun to interact with his fears. I never became a full-on sadist with him. I did, however, intentionally not give him information, knowing it would drive him nuts. This is what he needed to face, though.

Hook had a very warm and caring personality. At times it was like pulling teeth trying to get down to his real issues and concerns. All the time, I knew I would be doing a piercing of his chest with hooks. This was chosen because of his issues with cuts and body alterations. Any severe impact was out of the question. He was too new and never had been on the receiving end of these types of activities.

I tell everyone I have no control over where they go or what happens to them during rites of passage. This is Hook's story of what happened on his journey. It took him about eight months to gather his thoughts and feelings before he put them down on paper for me.

Who I am today is the result of thousands of decisions that I have made – a direct line stretching back through time and place to before I was born. Every decision was based on the outcome of the previous ones.

So what decisions led me to have my flesh pierced with hooks on that Sunday in December?

At 37 I had entered a period of change that at times seemed to be moving at warp speed. It was sometimes frightening, sometimes exhilarating, always new. Part of this change was an extreme awareness of my physicality, often to the point of distraction.

Now, perhaps a little background might be useful.

It was during preparatory discussions surrounding FifthAngel's upcoming Hawaii workshop (the workshop was held December, 2004) that I spoke of my fears to him. We talked about my fears and FifthAngel helped me examine them for proof of substance. My fears were surrounding my mortality.

I understood that FifthAngel had a gift for helping people face their fears, and so I asked him if he would help me face mine. I told him I wanted to die so that I would no longer fear death. FifthAngel agreed that he would help me. (Metaphorically of course.) At this point I put myself in his hands and allowed that whatever work he felt was best would be what would happen. He asked if I would be willing to have the work done in front of other people so that it could be part of a class. I told him that that was fine as I figured fairly soon into the work I would not care whether there was anyone or not. Little did I know.

He was rather vague as to what the work would be except to say that he was leaning towards piercing work. He also said that since we had not ever met in person, he would not make a final decision until we had some time to spend together face-to-face.

My wife was very supportive in whatever I needed to do to face my fears. It was important to have her support, although at the time and for a while after the weekend she simply could not understand what had happened.

Time passed and the weekend for the workshops came, and I found myself on Oahu. Friday and Saturday's activities went well and were very intriguing. I didn't think too much about Sunday's work until I got up that morning. All weekend FifthAngel had been as vague as he had been on the phone about what was going to happen on Sunday. I became more and more nervous as the morning passed and we were closer to leaving for the pre-workshop potluck. We arrived at the location, and I immediately headed for the woods for some solitude and to look for a possible place for the work to be done. I returned more grounded and ready for lunch. After lunch I asked FifthAngel about the location of the work. No, actually what I asked about was how he thought things were going. The question was the lead-in to the actual question, which was: will the work happen here or is it possible to have it up in the woods? The second question never got asked, as very quickly FifthAngel was off again prepping for the class.

The class was on Piercing for Spirituality, a title that intrigued me from the first time I saw it on his web site. He first covered safety. FifthAngel passed around needles and hooks and a volunteer was brought in to show placement and for some hands-on practice. After the demo was over, FifthAngel told me it was time to get ready. At this point my fear started to increase. I called a friend who had been sitting outside and asked her to come inside for support. FifthAngel instructed me to lean back against a massage table and pull off my shirt. I realized I had to go pee and told him so. He looked a little annoyed and said, "You'd better be quick." I came back and got in position leaning against the table. At this point he said that if I did meditation, it would be a good time to start. I closed my eyes, and started to concentrate on my breath. A wave of fear overtook me and I had an urge to run. At that point I remembered reading an essay that FifthAngel had sent me written by a woman who had worked with FifthAngel a couple of years back. Something she wrote really stuck with me – that during her work with him she reminded herself that she had asked for this. That thought allowed my fear to pass over and through me and kept me in place to receive the work.

FifthAngel used full sterile technique. The initial piercing was to be done with a piercing needle, followed by the 12-gauge salmon hook that he had prepared and sterilized. The sites were between the nipple and the collarbone about an inch and a half off the centerline. He pierced my left chest first. My breathing was slow and even and I knew that he would wait until I began to exhale. I don't know if he telegraphed his intentions unconsciously or if I was just tuned in, but I knew before he was going to push the needle through. He pushed the needle in, and I pushed my breath out, and it was done. I began to laugh and cry. It didn't hurt as much as I had feared and I had pushed past the barrier. He followed the needle with the hook and the first side was done. The right side was done the same as the left. I remember that one side was slightly more painful than the other, but at this point I don't remember which.

FifthAngel now had me stand up, move forward, and had the table moved out of the way. He had me move back so that I was directly underneath a block and tackle that was attached to the roof. He ran a cord through the eyes of both the hooks and tied the ends off. To the center of this loop he attached a line from the block. He took up the line until the cord had started to pull the hooks upwards. At this point a phrase that came into my mind was: "Time to go home." FifthAngel gradually started placing tension on the hooks. I felt myself instinctively rising up to reduce the tension. FifthAngel stopped and I settled back down onto the hooks. It was somewhat uncomfortable but not unbearably so. This pattern was repeated at intervals: FifthAngel would pull up; I would follow and then settle back down.

The entire time I had my eyes closed. In the beginning I didn't notice anything unusual about what I saw. Normally when I close my eyes it is primarily dark with some lighter color variations thrown in, mostly yellow. After awhile I began to notice what I was seeing was mostly purple with some white thrown in. At the time I didn't think anything of it.

One thing I did seem to notice was the people in the room talking. At least that's what it seemed like, people talking quietly, just at the edge of hearing. I didn't pay attention to what they were saying because I was focused on my breathing and on the hooks. I do have to admit that the thought crossed my mind: "Hmmm ... people are talking during the demo. That's a little unusual, and perhaps a little inconsiderate." It wasn't enough to make me open my eyes or pull me completely from where I was at, but it did cross my mind.

After what seemed like three or four minutes I began to feel lightheaded and as if I was going to pass out. I later found out that the time had been closer to ten minutes. I intensified my concentration on my breath, in the hopes that it would pass. It became clear that it wasn't going to, and so I opened my eyes and turned to FifthAngel. I told him I felt as if I was going to pass out. He immediately released the tension on the line, and I sank to my knees. I don't recall him moving, but as I slumped forward on my knees FifthAngel was in front of me, and as my forehead touched his chest his arms closed around me. The instant my forehead touched his chest the purple and white behind my eyes was instantaneously replaced with jet-black. I began to sob. After awhile the emotion passed and I opened my eyes. FifthAngel asked me if I was okay, and I said yes. He asked me if I wanted to leave the hooks in, and I said yes. He helped me to a chair and I sat down to watch the rest of the afternoon's workshop.

At this point I was in a bit of a daze. I watched the rest of the class from a bit of a distant perspective. Humorously enough, at one point a gentleman came up and asked me with a straight face: "Did it hurt?" I couldn't even answer. After about an hour the workshop was finished and FifthAngel asked me if I was ready to have the hooks taken out. I said yes. The removal was anti-climactic, and in fact one side did not even bleed.

The group began putting away chairs and putting the house back in order. I made a rather feeble attempt at being part of it all, but the fact of the matter was that I was gone. I had wisely given away the keys to the rental car to a friend before things started because I knew I wasn't going to be able to drive. Another friend gave me a ride home in her Miata. The ride was like nothing I had experienced before. The top was down, and I soaked in everything as we passed. I remember the trees and vegetation most of all. We went across the H3 and I can still see the plants as we entered the tunnel. As a note: when it comes to driving I like to be in control. I drive virtually any time I'm in a car. I chauffeur for my wife. When we go out with friends I offer to drive.

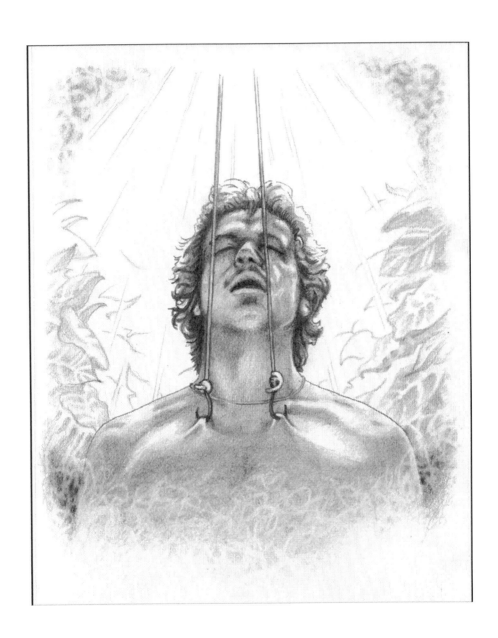

You get the picture. Here I was riding along with someone I'd never driven with before. I was in the passenger seat, in what is possibly one of the smallest cars on the road and at sixty plus miles an hour we are tailgating and swapping lanes like Mario Andretti. I had no fear. Normally this would have freaked me out. But I had no fear. Same thing for the plane ride home: no fear. This was the beginning of unintended/unexpected consequences.

We reached my friend's home and I decided I would like to just sit in the car. Fair enough. My friend went inside, and I sat in the sun with my eyes closed. I could've sat there for hours, but soon enough FifthAngel and the others showed up in the rental car, fresh from chasing parked cars.

The rest of the evening was mostly a blur. I do remember speaking to my wife on the phone. She was afraid. She knew I was different, but not sure in what way. This scared and unsettled her – more unintended consequences. I told her everything would be okay and that I would see her the next night. She seemed rattled but accepted my word that it would be okay.

The next day I had the opportunity to debrief with FifthAngel. One of the most interesting things that I found out in this conversation was concerning what I thought was people talking while I was on the hooks. It turns out that in fact nobody was talking. Well then just who was? If I'd known that it wasn't people in the room, I would've listened harder.

An interesting side note: I relayed this story to a friend of mine, and I knew as soon as I said it what his thoughts were. I asked him and he confirmed that I was correct. Demonic possession. Oh, well, different strokes for different folks. We have since had further discussions and he understands a lot more than I ever expected.

This is the end of my recollections of what happened during the weekend. However, it certainly is not the end. The choices I made and the things that happened during that week in Oahu have continued to reverberate in my life. Directly and indirectly several times a week it comes into my consciousness. It has become part of the lexicon that my wife and I share. The hooks and the cord hang from my rearview mirror and I see them on a daily basis. That is why I feel like I should continue and share with you as best I can the ripples that have spread out from that day.

As soon as I got off the plane, my wife knew I was different, even more so than on the phone. Quickly I realized what she was picking up on. I went to Oahu to face and deal with my fears surrounding my physicality. I lost those fears at least for a while, but what I didn't realize is that I had lost all of the rest of them as well. I was no longer afraid of my wife. If you had shown me that sentence the week before, I would've said, "What the hell do you mean, afraid of my wife?" I was unaware of the fact that I was afraid of her. I was unaware of the fact that I was afraid of my parents. I was unaware of the fact that I was afraid of my friends. I was unaware of the fact that I was afraid of my business contacts. I went to Oahu because I was afraid of death, and I was afraid of my body. I came back realizing I had been afraid of life. I've since realized how and where a great many of those fears came from, and how lessons learned as a child remained unwanted behaviors three decades later.

I have since realized that at a very young age I learned that if I did not make everyone happy, they would take their love away. I have spent my entire life in fear that if I did not make everyone happy, they would remove their love/friendship. Unintended consequences.

The day after I came back I attempted to go to work. As soon as I came on the job site my friend and business partner looked at me and smiled. He said, "You're different." I said, "I know." He summed the change up in one word: "stronger." I did not tell him for a couple of weeks what happened, but he knew something had changed while I was off island. Very quickly I realized that work was not the place that I wanted to be. It held absolutely no interest. Fortunately I work for myself, and I was able to take the entire month off.

I needed it. Within two days I was on the phone with FifthAngel, crying and asking if it was crazy that I wanted to be back up on those hooks – back in the clarity and the purity. I was no longer afraid, but I was also no longer fully in this world. It took me two or three weeks before my appetite came back. Immediately following the event I had little appetite. I did not force myself and therefore my intake dropped drastically. Looking back I realize that it was a way of keeping myself in that altered state.

Before the work FifthAngel had me read an essay by a friend of his named Travis. At the end of Travis's essay he said he needed two days by himself. If you are considering doing work of this type, listen to what Travis has to say. I would say two days is a bare minimum – more time if you can get it.

It took two weeks before my wife and I felt comfortable around each other again. I was no longer afraid of her, and that scared her tremendously. At first glance that may sound like a pretty strange sentence, but what it really means is that my emotional connection/entanglement had been broken, and she was unsure of whether we would ever be reconnected. I knew she was afraid, but her emotions seemed almost peripheral to me. Breaking the entanglements in the end allowed it to be rebuilt on a cleaner level.

The same was true with my mother. I did not bite when she tried to pull my strings. This freaked her out.

This all may sound pretty intense, but I guess that's because it was. Having said that, I would not change a moment of it, but it was a much larger decision than I knew at the time. I am stronger for it.

I don't want to make it sound like a magic bullet. A number of the fears of all types that I had before the work have returned. They haven't returned with the same quality that they had before. The work has allowed me to look at them differently, more detached. My life has changed in a number of ways since then, and I feel that the work that I did with FifthAngel has had an effect to some degree on all of it.

Something which has stayed with me is faith. I have not had faith for a long time. When I say faith I mean a feeling of connection, a feeling of being part of something greater. A sense that when it is all done, I will be okay. I still have fear surrounding death, but it seems to be around the event itself, not about what comes after it – letting go, the loss of control, not the backside.

If given a chance, would I do it again? It would have to be the right place and time, but yes, I think I would. Only next time I would want to follow in Travis's footsteps and fly.

Now where did I put my red cape?

Finding Release Beyond the Pain
by Sherrye Segura

My relationship with Sherrye is very different from any of my others. Whereas Leslie is my consensual slave, Sherrye is more of a girlfriend. She is by no means a bottom for heavy scenes on a regular basis. More to the point, she does not bottom all that much period. To say she bottoms to me would really be stretching it. What we have is sadistic sex. Sherrye is not submissive to me, although she will perform acts of kindness and helpfulness. But ask her to lick my boots or get spanked, and I think one of my boots would come flying back at me. Okay, I think she is too nice to really do something like that, but you get the point, I'm sure.

It is true that I almost never ask people to scene. Yes, there are those times when a bottom is fumbling with words in an attempt to ask me for a scene. It is then that I will assist a bit and ask them to lessen their strain. With Sherrye though, the feeling was there and I reluctantly asked her. I thought to myself, "This could be very dangerous." – dangerous in the sense that I knew my emotions would be involved, maybe too involved.

When she helped me with my class, which you will read about, I felt the potential for something deeper with her. Sure I could try and flip the switch once again, but I didn't want to, not with Sherrye.

During my class I had to step back, literally, because my sadism was overpowering me. My head was flooded with images of her and me. Her partner and my entire class were watching. Rather than act on instinct, I chose to have Sherrye's partner step in and take over for me. That was when I fully realized the potential if she and I ever scened together. We both had significant others. My fear was of their not understanding. With Sherrye, I felt that there was potential for a longer lasting relationship. What we had to explore could not be done in one scene or even a weekend. I had not felt this way before, other than with my slave.

Throwing my heart out on the line, Sherrye did say yes to my proposal to scene. It was a strange feeling, the possibility of rejection from someone I really wanted to scene with in a very sexual way. Life would have gone on if she had said no, though. I prepared my slave as well as possible for the type of scene I felt it would be. The four of us sat and talked about what might happen. These events took place at Camp Crucible, an event where all four of us were well known. We have many friends who attend Camp with us. Knowing we would be turning some heads by scening together, there was no way to prepare our friends and the potential rumor mill that might turn up. But these sorts of things happen when people do sexual scenes in public. Those issues were discussed, but would never have been a reason for Sherrye and I not to scene.

Our interactions at Camp that year led to my first polyamorous relationship. Now "first" does not mean there will be more. And as I write this, Sherrye and I continue to explore sadistic sex. Sure, I push her beyond her limits into new areas. It is a natural progression to do so. Because there is love with her beyond the normal care I have for my partners, Sherrye is not a bottom to me; she is more than that. While reading this introduction, I hope you realize that Sherrye is not a masochist. She is not one to say she likes painful sex. But each time the sex is about consensual sadism. I guess she puts up with it because she loves me.

A month or two prior to Camp, FifthAngel did a workshop on blood play and cupping at The Crucible. After becoming enthralled and extremely turned on by his demonstration, I knew that I had to ask for a tutorial to learn as much as I could. I have been fascinated and drawn to blood play for a long time because of the spiritual and bonding aspects, but the risks of such play and fear of the unknown, along with my inexperience, had kept me from pursuing my desires.

I remember watching the blood drip from an I.V. tube onto his demo bottom and imagining myself in her position. A hunger ached in the pit of my stomach and I felt myself get wet. With my heart pounding in my ears and the heat rising from my face, I knew that the desire had become a need I had to fulfill. Unfortunately, I had little opportunity to speak with him about further details or get him to teach me because I was working that night, but he mentioned his workshop at Camp and the possibility of showing me then. So I placed that as a priority among must-attend presentations since I would be on staff again.

When I went to Camp Crucible 2005 it started out as a need to get away and clear my head. I was not only burned out and run down from work but also from basic everyday issues. So Camp was the perfect opportunity to find that peace of mind.

As a staff member of The Crucible and most of the events sponsored by the club for the past four years, I knew that, even though we worked non-stop and rarely got time to enjoy the pleasures and free time that our attendees did, just being in a different environment amongst leather family and friends away from the stress would help. However, Camp Crucible turned out to be very different for me that year and started a new chapter in my life – one that I never expected…

As we came into the dungeon affectionately named "Heaven," FifthAngel had already started explaining different methods of blood play. We sat down near the back trying not to disturb the class and I watched intently and tried to soak in as much as possible. When he asked for volunteers to demonstrate capillary bleeding, my partner Stephen raised his hand and offered to be the demo bottom since he had never experienced it. We all chuckled at the faces that he made while FifthAngel took his time inflicting the pain that he enjoyed so much as he went through the different methods and tools of how to do it.

My mouth watered as I watched the blood seep down his arm. After FifthAngel was finished and had cleaned him up and applied a bandage to his deltoid area, Stephen came and took his place beside me and revealed his small but still bleeding wounds to me. I instinctively took his arm and ran my tongue along the wet and dried streaks until they all but disappeared, getting caught up in the sweet coppery taste. It seemed I was lost in the moment and then finally came back to listening to what was being said.

After cleaning up and passing around a few instruments to view, FifthAngel proceeded to explain his next demonstration and asked who had not experienced venous catheters before and asked for volunteers. I raised my hand and then he looked right at me and said my name, and without a second thought I stood up, kissed Stephen, and went up to the front. FifthAngel asked me to remove anything that I didn't want blood on and I felt hesitation take hold of me for just a moment. As much as I wanted to experience this and learn from him, I was afraid of how I was going to react.

I took my clothes off and climbed up on the table after a few whistles and comments from our friends who were present and then took a deep breath. Not only was I nervous about what he was going to do, but being in front of everyone caused a slight bit of embarrassment as well. Leslie brought him a new pair of gloves and he asked me if there were any bloodborne diseases that he should know about and I answered no.

After a few minutes of him talking he looked at my arms and veins and decided that he would put the catheter in my left arm. He had placed a tourniquet on my upper arm following standard medical technique and then I felt a slight twinge of pain as he slipped the needle in quickly and effectively after having to bypass a turn in the vein. He proceeded to explain further and then moved on to placing a venous tube onto the catheter after I had bled out for a few moments, showing how to open and close it.

The catheter was taped down to my arm and then he came around to the other side and the room got quiet as he took the tube in his hands and explained how he enjoyed painting the body while doing blood play. He placed his hand on me and smiled while holding the tube up and then his smile turned to a serious and transcendent look as my blood flowed from the tube down the side of my body.

I remember feeling a warmth come over me, and it was almost like I could count every single drop that flowed out of my vein. My desire and need to feed grew stronger with each bloody line I felt him make on my skin and I was incredibly excited. I could feel my body move and arch slightly in reaction to what was happening. My right arm moved above my head and grasped my hair as he brought the tube up to my neck and across my chin.

It brought goose bumps to the back of my neck as it disappeared beneath my head and then, as I felt it over my lips, my mouth opened and my tongue slowly searched for what I needed. The few steady streams into my mouth were enough to bring me close to orgasm and so delicious, but it wasn't enough to quench my thirst or the hunger that lingered in my gut. I wanted more but he moved down my neck again, and the wetness from my sex flowed onto the sheet beneath me.

He stopped and asked if I was ok and then asked if I was sure I had never done this before and laughed. I shook my head slowly no, having a hard time answering and he explained that some people enjoy eating their own blood just as I did and mentioned his slave Leslie as well. I looked at Leslie and smiled because I had been witness to this a few times and had seen how much she enjoyed feeding on her own blood.

My head returned to center position and I could feel myself letting go, but in a realm that I had never experienced before. He had his hand on me and it was warm even through the latex glove. I could feel the stream of blood he released seep through the crevice of the already wet folds between my legs and he became locked into what he was doing as he watched the blood continue to flow and my body react to the attention it was receiving.

I could feel the energy that surrounded us become stronger and desired him to touch me. The need to have that sexual ache subside that had grown so intensely was almost as large as the hunger I had for my own blood. After what seemed like only a moment stuck in time he cleared his throat and I could hear the nervousness and sexual excitement in his voice as he handed the tube to Stephen and said, "You better take this."

I felt Stephen lean over me and continue to stream the blood over me for a few minutes, enjoying feeling the warmth of his bare hands as he ran them over my bloody body tracing patterns and smearing it into my skin. FifthAngel relieved him of the tube and Stephen continued to lick blood from me and kiss me. The energy had changed and I could feel his hesitance during the bloodletting, his concern for me taking over.

He had been worried about the amount of blood I had lost and asked FifthAngel about it. I enjoyed his attention and the intimacy of sharing that with him, but it seemed my need and desire for blood play was a bit stronger and more tolerant for the experience at the time than his seemed to be. He had difficulty feeling secure and enjoying it because of his lack of knowledge. I had no worries and completely trusted FifthAngel and did not want it to end so soon. I could have lain there and been bled to death and not thought twice about it. I wanted more. I needed more.

FifthAngel had taken the catheter out and told me to drink something and also warned me of the possibility of feeling weak and faint for a while. Stephen helped me sit up and I still felt very disoriented. I struggled to figure how I was going to get off the table without getting blood all over the place, my brain being a little slow in solving that problem, and Stephen saw my distress.

He bent down and picked me up off the table very much like a fairytale groom with his bride and, wrapped up securely in the stretcher sheet, I wrapped my arms around his neck. Leslie handed me my clothes and he turned to face the few people applauding and making sweet comments on his efforts to care for me.

Stephen carried me all the way up to our cabin that was on the hill next to the dungeon even after me telling him that I was fine to walk. He deposited me in the shower and he and our submissive helped clean me up and then he disappeared from the cabin. I took a few minutes to myself and changed, fighting with the emotion that started coming out full force.

A lot of things are hazy so I am not sure I am taking them into account correctly as far as events unfolding, but I was well aware of the profound effect on me afterwards. My lust for blood was awakened and I knew for certain that this was only the beginning. I was also suffering a great deal of confusion from the disconnection from my partner but this was not something that had been unusual over the past couple of years. Our relationship had suffered a great many problems regarding play and his distance and distraction was just another common occurrence.

The one person who had initially known of my desire for blood was now seemingly unaware of the aftercare and intimacy that I needed and the profound effect that it had on me and I was hurt a great deal. I had a hard time keeping the tears at bay, still feeling very emotional and foggy from what I had been through, but decided that

I also needed to thank FifthAngel and Leslie for the experience and time they took with me. So after I dressed I headed back down to the dungeon alone to give them both my thanks.

FifthAngel was immersed in a conversation so I shared my gratitude with Leslie and told her I would thank FifthAngel later when I had a chance to speak to him personally.

That night after dinner Stephen and I discussed what had happened during and after the demonstration. We both talked about the lack of communication that had happened and the issue was resolved. We went to our cabin and also talked about my desire to do a blood bonding while we got dressed for the night's activities. When we entered the dungeon we saw FifthAngel with Leslie and a few other people and I went over to him and finally told him thank you and gave them both a hug.

FifthAngel grabbed my arm and asked how it felt while he pushed into my vein and I winced telling him it felt a little sore but it was fine and then showed him the mark that had bruised slightly. I could see the tiny glimmer in his eyes as I winced, very aware of the fact that he wanted to inflict more pain when he giggled at my reaction. We chatted for a few moments and I asked if he could help with the scene that we wanted to do and he said that he had a couple of scenes but would be in the dungeon until late and to come and get him when we were ready. I was happy that he had agreed to help and be there for safety measures and to help guide us through the scene.

Stephen and I had met FifthAngel and Leslie about three years ago, so we both knew them but had not had a real chance to culminate in more than a friendly acquaintance. Since they did not live in the
D.C. area, the most we saw them or spoke to them was either through their classes, at big events, or at the club. So it was pleasant to be able to spend some time with them and get to know them a little better.

I had gained a certain respect for FifthAngel and his play style over the years by attending a few of his workshops and having the opportunity to watch him play a couple of times but had no desire to ever bottom to him. He scared me. In my mind his style of play was that of the extreme - a type of play filled with pain and only something that a masochist or someone who had a need for pain or catharsis would enjoy. Only a true sadist would understand the method to his madness and I did not fit into any of those categories by my own personal desires of play as a bottom.

I trusted him without question because of his experience and medical background and the connections he made with his partners, but it still did not give me the desire to pursue any actual scene with him because I knew what he was capable of: many things which I never thought that I would ever be willing to put myself through or allow anyone else to do to me.

When we finally had a chance to get together that night and go through details of where and how things wanted to be done, FifthAngel took the lead of the scene. I started to undress myself but FifthAngel stopped me telling me that it was his job and part of making that connection before a scene. At this point, in the four years that I had been with Stephen, no other man had shared the intimacy of undressing me, so it made me quite nervous to have FifthAngel do this and very awkward when he stopped me from helping him.

He was careful and kept eye contact and talked to me until it came down to my corset and garters which he tried to take off but had no idea where to start. So I ended up removing them myself. The small moment of humor over his frustration was a relief I appreciated since I could feel that same energy there again as I did earlier during the demonstration. It made me wonder if it was just this new experience or if that connection or sexual attraction was as strong as my stomach was telling me.

I stood there for a few minutes and my body began to shake. Between being nervous and the cold draft in the dungeon, I had a hard time keeping warm. They moved the heater over to try and warm me up and then I climbed onto the table. I was afraid that because of my body tremors I was not going to be able to stay still enough for FifthAngel to place a needle in me and I could see his concern for my shaking.

FifthAngel asked me if I had ever experienced needles before, and I said yes so he decided to do some play piercing to get my adrenaline going. I remember my shaking calming down after he placed two needles through my skin. He used a larger gauge and the slight pain was a welcome and warming relief as I felt the rush of adrenaline go through my body.

While doing the scene, FifthAngel tried to give instructions to my partner Stephen and answer questions, but I was not achieving the headspace that I needed, so again he took the lead and took measures to put me where I needed to be. A lot of what happened after that is still unclear except for certain things that linger in my head.

I remember lying there and being tied to the frame that was over the table by the needles in my chest and feeling my skin stretch every time I arched or trembled with an orgasm, not being able to move very far. I could feel the adrenaline and slight twinges of pain that made me want more every time they played with the needles under my flesh until it became too intense and I would try to melt into the table.

I recall Stephen and our submissive ayla feeding from the blood that covered my body and sharing in it myself with them from their lips or fingers, enjoying their attention as they touched me. And I remember FifthAngel pulling out a needle from the jugular vein in my neck that I couldn't recall him placing in me. I orgasmed continuously for a long time without any direct attention to my womanhood and remember hearing my release echo back to me even before my partner ensued direct stimulation.

I also remember this incredible connection that flowed between FifthAngel and me even though he did not take part in sharing my blood. It was strong enough to almost touch. I could feel it as he touched me and maintained verbal contact with me, asking me to cum for him. The sexual tension and need to kiss each other were there, but he did not overstep any boundaries because we had not spoken about it beforehand. His voice was what kept me grounded and safe and increased my sexual need even more as he whispered in my ear.

I had sometime in the process of his playing with the needles in my chest grabbed hold of his cock without a thought. I suppose subconsciously I used my hold on him as a method to keep him near me and to let him know when the pain became too intense when they played with the needles buried in my chest. It was way out of character for me to touch someone sexually without asking, and he seemed to take pleasure in reminding me of that incident the next day when it caused me a bit of embarrassment. So I apologized after he commented on my grip.

The next day I ran into FifthAngel again and we discussed how I felt. He had wrapped his arms around my neck and stood behind me as he asked if I would be interested in playing with him one on one, his question almost shy and boyishly charming. It was surprising to hear him ask because FifthAngel is not typically the one to ask if someone wants to play. Usually he plays with his slave or his day is full from people asking him to play or demonstrate his teachings. So I found it quite irresistible after my previous experiences with him and also very sweet in the way he approached me about it, not expecting that type of response from him.

I mentioned FifthAngel's request to my partner Stephen after I had thought about it for a while and then told him that I would like to play with him. Stephen, FifthAngel, his slave Leslie, and I sat down and had a discussion about both of our relationships and play. We discussed the obvious attraction and connection that he had to me and talked about the likelihood of it becoming very sexual.

Each of us was very honest and open about our own feelings and opinions of FifthAngel and me playing and the communication and negotiation went very well. Sitting back and listening I knew that the connection that I had felt was there for him, too, and was a resolution to the confusion I had felt the day before.

But now my concern was turned into a debate within myself whether I could handle playing with FifthAngel and why I wanted to even though the decision for me to play with him had already been made. My instinct knew that this scene was not going to be like any other scene I had been involved in before and told me that the possibility of my becoming prey to a larger animal than myself was highly likely. I knew that he would push me to my furthest extent physically, mentally, and emotionally and the red flags came out.

I began to worry about those walls that I had so securely built within myself and wondered if this was the right decision for me since it had been so long since I had actually played, since I am not a person who enjoys pain for pain's sake and agreeing to play with a sadist was completely confusing to me and I had to ask myself if I had lost my mind.

I feared him, and my imagination of what was going to transpire and the pain I was going to be put through did not help my nervousness throughout the day. But through all of this, in the back of my mind I was excited. I was turned on by that fear, and that sexual tension and attraction between the two of us.

It was a place that I had never been before, one where I had never allowed anyone to go. I had a personal need to be broken down, piece by piece, to gain the strength and knowledge that I could face whatever it was that he was going to put me through and survive. To allow myself to let go for a while and hopefully learn that my submissive side really was still there.

But even through the fear, there was a piece of me that knew that I trusted him, and that I trusted my life in his hands. He had proven that to me the day before when he had been my lifeline and had controlled the amount of blood that I shed as well as my mental state. He had the ability to read me and get through to me with ease, and that made me feel secure.

Because of the demo and then the scene I had done the night before, my arms and chest and neck were already covered in bruises where I had been pierced with needles, and my puncture wounds were sore. I knew that because I bruised so easily and it had been a long time since I had played that there would be many more to come.

When it was time for me to meet FifthAngel for our scene, I went in with our submissive and a close friend. Stephen had stayed behind, telling me he would arrive in a bit, and I knew he had already started having difficulty with jealousy and doubts and he needed time alone to get a hold of himself.

It was cold outside and in the dungeon, but FifthAngel had moved the heater close to the corner that he had chosen to play in. There were several wrestling mats lined up and the bondage chair was against the wall and immediately my mind began to race and my heart thudded in my chest wondering what he had planned on doing.

I saw Leslie and hugged her and we spoke for a few minutes. She told me that she had made a place for her and Stephen to cuddle and sit together while FifthAngel and I played and that was comforting. I thanked her for being so concerned with Stephen and wanting to share time with him during our scene.

I knew that this was not going to be easy on him since it was the first time since we had been together that I had requested to have someone else top me in an actual scene other than instruction, and that it would do him good not to be alone. My own concern grew as I stood there, wondering if he was going to be able to watch me play with someone else after the difficulties we had experienced over the past few years. But I knew that I had to do this for me, and it was a step in the right direction. I needed this.

I was standing there warming up my hands, and FifthAngel came over to me and warmed up his hands also. He took my hands in his and blew on them and then asked me if I was ready. I nervously laughed and told him no. He looked at me and asked why and I could feel the heat come to my face and I told him that I was afraid and nervous.

I told him that he made me nervous because I knew what he was capable of. He laughed and then asked me if I trusted him and I said yes. He took me by the hands and pulled me to him and asked if there was anything that I did not want him to do or anywhere I did not want him to touch me. The only request that I made was that there be no visible marks other than what I had already because I had to go back to work and would have my children the following weekend. I certainly did not want to look like I had been in a car wreck when my children saw me, and I was already half way there.

He took my hand and put it on his chest and then kissed me. He then told me that he had one rule that I had to follow. I would not be allowed to touch him at all during the scene. Now this may not seem very hard for some people but for me this was like telling me I could not breathe.

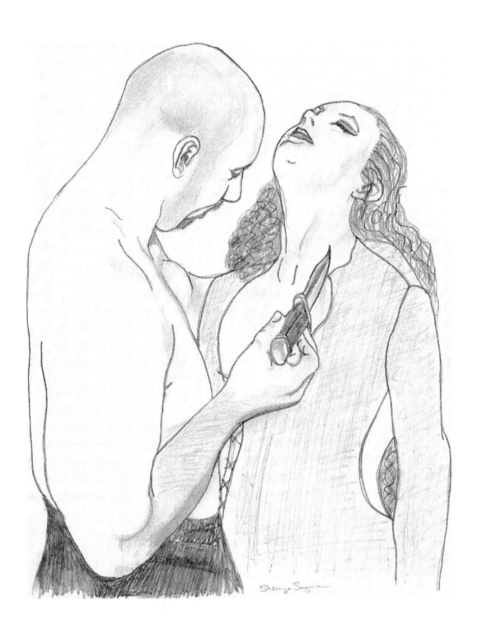

I am a very hands-on person and I enjoy that contact and he knew this so he used this against me. His voice was very stern and very serious and I knew that if I made the mistake of disobeying him that I would pay for it.

He took me by the hand and led me to the middle of the mat and stood in front of me. He pulled me closer into him and then kissed me again and pressed his forehead to mine. I could feel that energy flowing between the two of us and I was consumed by it. I could feel his heart beating against my chest and mine pounding against his. I was already wet.

My eyes were closed and I felt the sharp tip of a blade trace the features of my face from my forehead to my lips and a moan escaped my lips. He had found another way to get inside my head and it was through my love of knives. It helped me forget about my nervousness.

He undressed me, removing the top half of my dress after debating whether or not to cut it off me, and then got down on his knees in front of me and proceeded to remove my shoes. I became unbalanced at this point trying to stay steady without touching him and he held me up to keep me from falling. He placed my hands on his shoulder to keep me still.

After placing my shoes to the side, he bit into my left side and I hollered out, balling my hands into fists so I wouldn't touch him, and he rose up once again. He looked at me and placed his hands in my hair and pulled my head back and asked if I wanted to hit him and I replied no.

Using the knife once again, he used the point of the blade to open my mouth where he placed pressure on the middle of my tongue until my mouth was completely opened. He then took the blade and traced the vein in my neck and down the middle of my chest and then took the knife and threw it to the side of the mat.

He finished undressing me and I stood there completely naked for a moment and he grabbed me by both of my forearms, applying pressure points and brought me to my knees immediately in front of him. I had made the mistake of touching him without thought and I knew it instantly. My eyes had locked with his and I knew that he could see my fear before he had put me on my knees. It happened so quickly and the pain had been so intense that it took me a moment before I knew what had happened. He still had a hold of my forearms and pulled my face into his groin where I could feel his hardness beneath his pants. I knew that it had turned him on to hear me scream out and to have me at his mercy; I just didn't realize that it had such an instantaneous effect on him before now.

After a moment he pulled me back up and then proceeded to pull my arm behind my back. Stepping behind me quickly and then pushing me down into the mat where he trapped my body underneath him. He applied pressure points to my neck and grabbed me by the hair, thrusting his groin into my ass where I could feel his hardness again. He then bit into my shoulder and I cried out and buried my nails into the mat beneath me.

I could feel my skin between his teeth and I thought for sure that he had opened me up, and I surprisingly wanted him to. I wanted him to tear open my flesh and draw blood, but at the same time I wanted him to stop. And then he bit into me again and I could hear the growls coming from him and it sparked yet another trigger, one deep within my soul – the same one that makes me crave the very fluid that flows through our bodies to keep us alive.

My inner animal reacted to this in such a way that it terrified me. This was my dark place, my secret, and he sensed it the first time he drew blood from me. It was a place I had touched on, but had never allowed myself to go further, even with my partner, for fear of losing control of my human and logical self. It was the loss of control that I feared and he knew it. He made me ejaculate and we were both covered in sweat and cum.

He continued to apply pressure points, bite me all over my body, and toss me around like I was nothing more than a rag doll, using his body to bring me to orgasm as he pressed and moved into me in various positions he put me in. His strength and skill were very obvious at this point and my attempts to pull away were useless. Now that I think about it as an afterthought, I am sure it looked very close to a rape scene without penetration of any kind, and it was very hard to tell we weren't having sex.

He started doing breath play and even when I couldn't breathe my body still processed it as pleasure. I had left puddle after puddle and it did not stop. I continued to react, sexually responding to his body, the pain, and the intensity. I tried fighting the pain and then finally submitted when I could no longer take it. He had pushed me past that wall and had taken me way beyond my own tolerance level and I prayed for him to stop, my own guttural growls turning to whimpers and tears.

He brought me to orgasm by using direct pressure points, his own body, and requests for me to cum until I was exhausted and felt I could not possibly cum again. He whispered in my ear how beautiful I was even through my tears, knowing that he saw everything beneath the surface.

I accepted the pain within myself and it became a way of giving back to him, sharing with him, and existing in a realm where everything and everyone else disappeared but the need and fire between us. It was a way of opening me up and seeing what was inside my soul. He placed my hand on him and wanted me to touch him and placed me on top of him. I was still afraid to disobey him and had a hard time allowing myself to do this. He had placed my face into his chest and I knew that he wanted me to respond with that by biting into him, but I still couldn't.

He released the beast inside me and accepted and wanted what I had been afraid to show anyone. It was brutal but honest, and the reality of not hiding anything between each other and facing everything together as it came was clear.

Even though FifthAngel was dressed from the waist down, our scene was intensely sexual and very primal. The only image that comes to mind to truly describe it is of two tigers mating. It is a force of nature, and an instinctual need that has the possibility of ending in death with one wrong move. That is what I felt when I was with him.

It was a connection so deep and so strong that I did not want it to end even when we were both exhausted and I knew I could not take any more. The pain eventually stopped but the intensity, hunger, and passion still continued as he held, touched, and kissed me, sharing few words between each other but seeing everything in each other's eyes. The hunger for more was something that we both knew would not stop after we ended our scene.

He finally laid his head down on my stomach and I stroked his head for a short while. My tears fell silently as I still felt the rawness and love coming from him. My instinct told me that he needed to know that I was ok. After awhile he climbed up beside me and covered me up, holding me close. We talked for a bit and he made me smile and laugh and we decided that it was time to bring Leslie and Stephen over to join us.

It was not an easy scene for many and caused a great deal of emotional turmoil for those around us. Our partners and those who were close, as well as some who were not, were confused and alarmed by the connection and energy between us. The emotion and sexual need was something that neither one of us had shared publicly with anyone but our partners. Everyone who had entered the dungeon could feel it and was drawn to it.

We had quite a bit of communicating to do before we left Camp regarding all parties because of the intensity and what transpired during that scene. FifthAngel and I were very honest with what we felt and were still feeling whenever we were around each other. It was hard not to be around each other without some sort of intimate contact. But in the end we all walked away with a new understanding and a closer relationship with each other and our partners because of it.

Since Camp, FifthAngel and I have developed a close relationship and bond. We have become friends; play partners, and lovers whenever time and distance allows us to be with each other. Our partners have supported us and we have been grateful for the opportunity of sharing this with each other. The love that I share with him is hard to describe, but we accept it for what it is. We do so without a need for labels and continue to explore and learn about one another freely without restraint and without fear of each other or ourselves.

Through our relationship I have learned that pain and suffering is what lets us know we are still alive and makes us aware of things that we take for granted everyday. It is a way to break down those subconscious walls and rediscover our true selves without hiding and without resistance. I understand now that I don't have to be a masochist to love or play with a sadist. It is not the pain that I enjoy; it is the pleasure and release beyond the pain, and the beast that lies within.

Living with a Sexual Sadist
by slave leslie

Some people have no idea what they are asking for when they approach me for various things. Case in point – after attending one of my MAsT: Jacksonville meetings, which lasted approximately two and a half hours, a boy inquired about being my slave. This was the first time I had ever met this boy and we had had very little one-on-one conversation during the meeting. He knew virtually nothing of my sexual habits or day-to-day activities as an owner. Yet, in a period of two and a half hours he felt he knew enough about me to ask me about being my slave. Well, that is not the whole truth. He felt compelled enough to send my slave an email asking if I would consider having him as a male slave.

That was not the first time someone acted on impulse without really understanding what he or she would be getting himself or herself into. Indeed, it is an honor and very flattering to receive such requests; they're just not well thought through. Sure, from the outside it can seem a fantasy come true, until some of those fantasies of fear and helplessness do come true. It is my hope that by reading what my slave has to say, people will learn it is not all that easy to live with a sadist day in and day out. When it comes down to it, many would only want such a life for a few hours at a time and then maybe only a couple times a month. What they may get in a scene at a public dungeon with a sadist may not be an accurate reflection of what everyday life would be like with him.

By no means am I attempting to scare you away from living with a person like myself. I am an educator; thus it is my hope that by reading what my slave has to say, it will allow you to look at sadism from a different point of view. It is my desire that you will learn that consenting to a sadist will cause you to possibly view yourself in a confusing way at first. You are not alone in thinking, "Why do I let them do this to me?" My answer would be, "If it feels right, then don't ask why." You do not need to know why a sunset is beautiful to you, just that it is.

I'm not what I'd consider a masochist – or at least if I am, I'm a pretty wimpy one. But when I say that to people who have watched scenes Master has done with me, they look at me in disbelief and ask, "If you don't like pain, why do you let him do that to you?"

There is no easy answer to that question for me. It's certainly not because I like pain for pain's sake. I don't transform it into pleasure and orgasm over and over. I don't float off into what I've heard others describe as subspace. No, I experience pain, and I endure it. Sometimes I fight it, sometimes I don't mind it so much, but I sure do feel it.

I always thought a masochist was someone who orgasmed to pain. I've learned there is a much larger definition – according to the DSM-IV, sexual masochism is diagnosed by meeting the criteria: "Over a period of at least 6 months, recurrent, intense sexually arousing fantasies, sexual urges, or behaviors involving the act (real, not simulated) of being humiliated, beaten, bound, or otherwise made to suffer." Well, that part fits me pretty well. Their criteria also states "The fantasies, sexual urges, or behaviors cause clinically significant distress or impairment in social, occupational, or other important areas of functioning." But I'm not experiencing any clinically significant distress from my chosen lifestyle, so it's not any kind of sexual disorder.

I suppose technically I could be called a masochist, because I masturbate to memories of our scenes afterward. But I still have reservations about accepting the label for myself due to its common BDSM definition – a bottom who is sexually aroused by pain. It's not memories of pain that I masturbate to, but more thoughts of fear and loss of control. Heck, the fantasies that I masturbate to would more often than not be fatal if brought into reality. I've learned to be very careful when expressing my desires to Master; he puts his own twists into my fantasies and, well, he *is* a sadist.

I have to confess I had no idea what a sadist was when I first met FifthAngel. I knew there were tops out there who were considered "heavy," and I'd scened with a few of them, but I always thought they only wanted to give pain that the bottom liked. I thought SM was always about the top and bottom getting off on pain and pleasure together.

So how did I, a wimpy pain bottom, end up as the 24/7 consensual slave of a sadist?

FifthAngel had been invited by Lolita Wolf to present at TES30. He told her he needed a demo bottom and sent her his specifications. She emailed me, stating, "Trust me, he's hot." So I told her I was interested and she put us in contact with each other. He and I shared about six weeks of emails, online chats, and phone conversations. It started with us discussing my ability to demo bottom for his workshops, but we quickly discovered that we complemented each other in many ways, and we began exploring the potential for a relationship. We agreed that I would be collared to him for the weekend of the event, and that we would share a hotel room. Yes, I know we were moving kind of fast, but for some deep reason, I trusted him.

In the few weeks we'd been getting to know each other, I'd shared some of my serial-killer type fantasies. I'd mentioned I liked breath control and fantasies of being helpless. FifthAngel told me that perhaps one night I might awaken to find duct tape covering my mouth, and he would bring one of my fantasies to life.

When we finally met in person, it wasn't long before we were scening. He'd started with a quick scene in the airport elevator (it was a short ride), and he did some fun pressure points on me during the drive to the hotel. He'd spilled a little of my blood in the shower, and we did a pressure point scene that left him writhing in pain on the floor (sorry, the hook broke and I ended up whacking him full force on the top of his head with my cuffed hands). We'd had a spanking scene in the dungeon that left me floating. He'd used his sword on pressure points all over my body, and that really hurt, but it wasn't too much pain for me to be able to process. These were scenes I really enjoyed and felt he did, too.

We went back to the hotel room after a fun night of scenes in the dungeon, and he took me by surprise with the duct tape while I was still awake. He was cheating already. Geez! But I was aroused as he pinned me to the bed with his body and pinched my nose closed. I squirmed against him and felt his hardness. After a few seconds, I shook my head and he released my nose. I was quite turned on. I was helpless in the arms of this very strong, very sexy man who wanted to make my fantasies come true. As he closed off my nose again, I was a little scared because I didn't think I could get away, but I didn't really want to, anyway. I knew he'd let me breathe again soon. But this time, when I shook my head, he didn't let go right away.

Okay, this wasn't quite what I expected. It started to hurt, and not in a good way. He let go before I could raise my hands to try to get away. Then he distracted me with some sensual touching and licking. Yummmm…

I flinched as his hand reached for my nose yet again, but I wasn't able to stop him from pinching my nostrils shut. I panicked and started to struggle in earnest. My body bucked under him, trying to flip him off me, while my hands tried to pull his from my nose. I was not at all successful. I truly couldn't get away from him. And I started to get really scared, not sexy scared.

Some part of my mind was rational enough to know he probably wouldn't kill me. People knew we were there together. But that didn't matter – my lungs were burning and it was a pain I had never felt before. But worse than the pain was the terror that there was nothing I could do to stop him. Nothing. My body was fighting to get away from the man holding my nose, and no matter how hard I struggled, I couldn't budge him.

I've felt helpless before. As a teenager, I was raped at knife-point by an acquaintance. I made the choice not to fight in that situation, but to just endure it and wait for it to be over. But that was the choice I made. This was completely different. This was a consensual scene of sadomasochism with someone I had feelings for, and who I believed cared about me.

So why was he still hurting me when I was struggling to get him to stop? All the other tops I'd scened with had stopped when I safeworded or signaled that I'd had enough.

When he finally let go of my nose, not much more than a minute could have passed. I wasn't anywhere close to passing out. I was pretty close to hysterics, though. He pulled the duct tape from my mouth and held me close. I was scared and angry and really confused. Nobody had ever been that mean to me before in a scene.

He distracted me with kisses and that led to sex and then we drifted off to sleep, exhausted. The rest of the weekend was pretty busy and I didn't have a lot of time to think about the emotional ramifications of FifthAngel pushing me so far with breath control.

Later, I must confess I eroticized the scene, as I recalled the yummy parts of it while masturbating. But I didn't really think about why he had kept going when I wanted him to stop. I thought maybe he just hadn't realized how bad it was for me.

Boy, was I clueless.

Our relationship progressed from that weekend collar to my moving from New Jersey to Florida to be FifthAngel's 24/7 live-in submissive, soon "promoted" to slave. Our scenes were frequent and often wonderful, but sometimes they would get a little too extreme for me to process well.

I remember at times wondering to myself: *Why the heck does he start so intensely? Warmup? He's supposed to be some really great top – so where the heck is my warmup? I can't handle most of what he really seems to like – I am doing everything I can to remember pain processing techniques like breathing and imagery – why can't I let go and make it not hurt?*

And after the pain, as I would curl up and bawl my eyes out on the floor, he wanted to have SEX! What the hell? I wanted to be cuddled and held and hear him say, "It's OK, I've got you, angel." About the last thing on my mind was sex.

And talking about sex, well, "regular" sex started off feeling good, but sometimes he'd go too deep, or too hard and it would hurt a bit. I've always liked it a little bit rough, but it kept getting more and more painful as time went on. And let's not even talk about anal sex … or fisting …

If it was so terrible, why did I stay? In so many ways, we were very compatible, and I was head-over-heels in love (still am, and hope always to be). I could handle a bit of pain and scary stuff here and there, and part of me got off emotionally on the "awful" stuff, and the sweet loving aftercare. But I still felt like I wasn't a very good bottom for him.

Sometimes while having sex, he'd mix in something that was "supposed" to be painful, like pressure points or biting, and I could use the sex part to enjoy the pain part a bit more. But mixing things like needles and sex just really confused me. It wasn't one thing or the other – sex or SM.

It took a couple of years and some hints from Master before I put it together that he *liked* it when sex hurt me – that he wasn't an insensitive clod; he caused pain on purpose. I mean, I knew he was being a sadist when he did SM activities on me, but I never quite connected SM and sex. Duh!

For a while after that, I started getting down on myself for not being a masochist. I thought he'd be more compatible with someone who liked the "awful" stuff he did – someone who could process what he wanted to do, instead of fight and cry. Sure, I'd heard Master say in his classes a few times that a masochist is a sadist's worst enemy, but it took a while until the light bulb finally came on in my head; I realized that my "failure" as a masochist makes us a very successful match as sadist and slave. Not only do I hate a lot of the things he likes to do, but my devotion to him as his slave provides me with intense satisfaction for being able to endure our scenes and feed his sadism.

Just when I got used to the fact that he's happier when I'm not enjoying myself, Master started working on "re-wiring" me by providing a bit of pain with my orgasms. I guess he thinks he can make a sexually-responsive masochist out of me. We'll see....

I do feel like Master has slowly seduced me into craving the pain and intensity of sadomasochism with my sex. At this point, I don't know what I'd do if he just laid me down gently on the bed and started tenderly making love to me.

Between Master and me, I think it is safe to say that sex is a scene and a scene is sex. Sometimes it's light and playful – a quick smack as I walk by is as good as a kiss to me. Occasionally it's a heavy beating that leaves bruises for weeks, or sex that leaves me so sore I start to cry when I see that he wants me again. Whether it's a flogger or his cock, it leads to the same place emotionally.

As the slave of a sadist, I do get my fair share of pain, both physical and emotional. But some people seem to think we're always having sadistic sex; sorry to disappoint you, but our life is not all about sex and pain. We have a very full life together, and we do love each other and are committed to each other for life. Master owns the house we live in; he goes off to work and I take care of the day-to-day chores: cooking, laundry, and all that "50s housewife" stuff. Not that we're married – Master and slave fit us a lot better than husband and wife. I am lucky enough to have a great job that lets me work at home, and a boss who is OK with the fact that I may end up on HBO some day.

There are actually a few areas of our life where he is not "FifthAngel" and not "Master." When we're SCUBA diving, rock climbing, or mountaineering, we are partners (sure, he's more experienced and stronger – but I'm just as responsible for our fun and safety).

But when he's in the mood to take out his sadism on me, there is no telling what form it will take. At home, painful sex often comes into play, but there are times Master will make it what I call an "official scene" in his dungeon. When we scene at events, most dungeons have rules against sex, so many of our public scenes don't involve intercourse.

I do occasionally scene with others, and sometimes I top. I, however, am not a sadist. I get off emotionally on the connection with my partners and the blood I draw from them, but it's not anything close to what I imagine Master feels.

When I bottom to trusted friends, scenes are usually a lot more playful and more equal in terms of both of us enjoying ourselves. I know I can take a lot, and I want my partner in the scene to go where he or she wants to go, but I have much less desire for heavy pain. I do enjoy different dynamics, such as being able to yell, "God damn it, Travis!" at the top of my lungs – not exactly something Master wants to hear from me (especially since his name is not Travis).

With others, there is still a desire to be pleasing and be of service, but it comes from a much different place than the "take anything you want from me" openness that I feel with Master.

For not being a masochist, I have taken a lot of pain from Master.

I've endured much that if I had known what he had in mind, I probably wouldn't have agreed to, because I didn't have enough faith in myself to know how strong the human body and spirit are. And on the other side of that endurance, Master has touched the deepest and most passionate places in my soul, and he's expanded my mind and spirituality in unimaginable ways.

There are many kinds of pain I've experienced with Master. Some I enjoy and process better than others. Some I crave, some I fight.

I've tried to convince him that I'm not Gumby, dammit, but he really seems to think I can do full splits and other little contortionist tricks during sex.

Master often takes me from behind. I think it may have as much to do with the scarification he has been designing on my back as it does the way my body feels to him. He can get awfully deep that way and it hurts a lot, but it's a really good hurt.

He's a biter, and there are times when I am afraid he will take a chunk out of my shoulder. At the same time, I yearn for him to bite deeply enough to draw blood. There are times when sex is very primitive and animalistic for both of us, and that's something I love. Though there was one time when Master was feeling like an animal and I wasn't, and he scared the heck out of me. He wrote about that in his chapter "What Are You Thinking?" I could feel that he wasn't Master any more, and I begged him to let me see his eyes, to see if he would come back.

Master is very skilled in the use of pressure points. During sex, he'll often use them to move me around or cause intense sensation. There are some points that are very erogenous, and others that cause a lot of pain. He likes to really mix them up and use them to bring up emotional responses, and also to position me in ways that please him. I love it when he uses pressure points on me, even when they are very painful.

Sometimes there's bondage, sometimes there's breath control. Sometimes I fight back a little bit and make it into a rape scene. But with all his skills and techniques from years of martial arts training and his own exploration of sadism, I know if I fight back a lot, he's just going to use more force, to the point where I'm not going to enjoy the experience at all – which in its own weird way provides a sense of satisfaction and release once it's over. It may have something to do with just surviving.

Master has flogged me until I felt the skin was peeling from my back (it wasn't). I felt like I couldn't stand it – not one more second, not one more stroke. But when he unchained my hands, I stood on my own and took more from him. He's used chain floggers on me until my back has bled. He's even drawn blood with nice soft suede floggers. He's pierced my back, removed the needles, and then flogged me. (It's really hard to get blood off white walls.)

He's beaten me with a shinai as I was bound to an X-frame in a public dungeon. Every blow caused me to scream and struggle to get away. If I hadn't been bound, I wouldn't have been there. As devoted to him as I am, I didn't think I'd be able to take it. But his taking that choice away from me showed me that my body is much stronger than I thought. I healed just fine.

Master has lit my skin on fire with many different implements – the most extreme being full-impact fire flogging – outside in fifty-degree weather. You know, I'm not sure which was worse, the fire itself or the bucket of cold water he poured over me before he got started, just to make sure my hair was still wet.

For some odd reason, and Master swears it's coincidental, he seems to like to bite my shoulders or flog me hard a couple of days before we have outdoor adventures. When we did a winter ascent of Mt. Hood, my back was black and blue, which made carrying a pack quite interesting.

He's pierced parts of me that really, really hurt – try having hub needles poked straight into the tips of your fingers and toes – yukky! I mean, that's just not right. Though he was smart enough to ask me, "If I pierce your clit hood while my cock is in your mouth, do you think you could refrain from biting me?"

In terms of emotionally "awful" sex, Master once looked at me with cold, dead eyes while he was fucking me painfully on the floor – leaving me crying, "I want Master!" He responded, "Your Master's not here." That was both terrifying and thrilling.

Master tied my hands behind my back, leaned me over the side of the tub, and poured pitchers of cold water over my face. I couldn't catch my breath, and I panicked. I completely lost track of who he was, and that I was in a consensual sadomasochistic scene with someone who loves me and would never harm me. That was probably the first time he triggered my fight or flight system. And when it's triggered and you can neither fight back nor fly away, it leads to a very painful place in the mind.

In bed one night, Master started to do some breath control along with sex. I ended up scratching his thighs in my effort to get away. He wrapped my hands in socks and Vetwrap, then continued fucking me and closing off my mouth and nose. The more I struggled, the worse it got. He told me I was only breathing when he chose to let me – it was up to him, out of my control. Again, I know he would never harm me, but I managed to forget that fact for a little while. But later … I still masturbate to memories of that scene at times.

For New Year's Eve one year, he pierced my back and suspended me from our dungeon hoist with huge salmon hooks. That was the first time I felt what I've heard others describe as an endorphin rush. Huge tingling waves of energy flowed up and down my back. Near the end of the suspension, our dog, Tenshi, came in and licked my feet. She's a great aftercare dog. Then Master took me to a hockey game. That was the real torture.

The next summer, he suspended me from a huge tree by the river at Camp Crucible. As Master hoisted me off the ground, the twanging of the rope made me hear music in my head. First was "Dueling Banjos" from the movie "Deliverance." Then came Earshot with "How much must I live through just to get away?" A lot, I guess.

Master said one day he will have sex with me when I'm suspended. That, I am strangely looking forward to.

Just before an early morning panel discussion at Spring in the South, Master started chewing on me, to the point where I was biting on my T-shirt to keep from screaming and disrupting other conversations in the area. He ended up stuffing most of my shirt into my mouth and most of my left breast into his. As he was winding down, he was very timidly interrupted by an event organizer, letting him know he really had to get up to the front of the room and join the panel. I snuggled on the floor with BD Bear (my birthday present from Master a few years ago) and brought myself back to earth.

We scened on a rooftop in New York City during Folsom Street East. Master had me hold a wakazashi (short sword) to my own throat as he helped me prepare for the female version of seppuku, ritual Japanese suicide. Of course he added his own touches to the ritual, including beating me with his shinai and using his sais on pressure points. And when I thought we were done and aftercare was beginning, he left me to drift by myself for a few moments. Our dear friend Barbara Nitke was photographing the scene and she told him, "FifthAngel, the light's just perfect." She swore later she meant "for aftercare," but he took it as a suggestion that he continue the scene. As he planted his sais in the palms of my hands, a fury came over me unlike anything I had felt toward him before. If I could have moved, I would have picked up Master, the man that I love more than anything and have devoted my life and heart to, and flung him over the edge of the roof.

Recently, we both had a rare day off at home with no plans. Master decided to give me a full day in the dungeon. He started the morning by suturing my mouth closed, which is something I love. It's very peaceful (for both of us) to take my words away. After the suturing, he hugged me and kissed me, said he loved me, and left the dungeon. He came back every hour or two, but he was emotionally detached. He would blindfold me and then chain me up in different uncomfortable positions and fuck the hell out of me. He'd cum, release me, give me a protein shake or a soda to suck through a straw, and leave. But he never said a word. That started to get to me – even though I know he loves me and that this day in the dungeon was a reward of sorts, it was still very disconcerting to be treated like dirt, like a prisoner, like I was useful for fucking but not for talking to. At one point he bound me face down on top of my cage, so that I could not move at all. Then he fucked me painfully yet again. That wasn't enough for him, so he reached around and held my nose. Because of the emotional distance he'd created with the blindfold and the silent treatment, I couldn't even remind myself that he loved me and would never harm me – I was really afraid of the pain he was causing me, and I believed he didn't care that he was hurting me. My panicked struggles did nothing to dislodge him, and I could feel how hard he was inside me. He let me breathe again and I had to focus on not crying, because if I did, my nose would stuff up and, with my mouth sutured shut, that would be a bad thing. He fucked me hard until he came, released my chains from the cage but left them on my hands, and left my blindfold on that time. I heard him leave the dungeon and I crawled into my cage to comfort myself. There's no use telling myself it's not real, it's just a scene, and my loving Master will be back. When it's happening, it feels very real. And pain hurts. The next time he came in, he fucked me again, then removed my sutures and had me suck his cock with my very sore and swollen lips. It was really hot, and I was so focused on pleasing him, being open to him, and loving him. I was also really enjoying being able to open my mouth after Master had kept it sutured closed for twelve hours. Then we snuggled on the floor and I felt so happy and so loved.

I do sometimes think about what the future will hold. Will Master need to cause more and more pain to remain sexually interested in me? Can I take what he wants to give me? Do I really want to have sex while being suspended by hooks in my back? Umm, well … I'll try anything once. (Okay, anything Master thinks is a good idea.)

It has been strange for me to accept that I am more of an emotional masochist, and that emotional pain enhances my physical endurance.

The times when Master combines both physical and emotional sadism have been some of the most powerful scenes I have endured. When he flogs me, and then takes a break to berate me for something I am having difficulty dealing with emotionally, and then flogs me even harder, something inside me lets go and does mute the pain. My anger at Master enables me to put the physical sensations aside, but at the cost of a great amount of emotional pain. I hate to be upset with him or disagree with him, and most of all I hate to fail him.

In his chapter "More Sadistic Techniques," Master wrote about a scene where he wanted me to think he was punishing me. Some background – I was unhappy with him because he was exploring something that pushed a lot of my "insecurity buttons." I felt like he wasn't taking my feelings into consideration. (Now, I know Master respects my rational feelings, but he's not going to rework his life to placate my irrational beliefs and expectations.)

When he took me up to the dungeon and brought out his escrima sticks, I was scared. I know how much they hurt. And being upset with Master and feeling like he was upset with me felt wrong – we were breaking "The Rules" by having a scene when we were angry! So he beat me – I use the term "beat," but please don't think it was an out-of-control wild-blows-landing-anywhere kicking-and-screaming beating. It was methodical and the blows landed very deliberately on my buttocks. Okay, so there was kicking and screaming, but it was on my part.

In between blows, he was asking me questions, and I was upset enough to pretty much blurt out whatever came into my mind – I have no idea if I was making sense or not – and now I'm glad to find out it didn't really matter. But the more upset I got, the more I focused on my emotional pain, and the more angry I got, the more determined I was to ignore that bastard and not give him the satisfaction of reacting to the physical pain.

There was a part of me deep inside that was really reveling in the darkness and rage that I was feeling. I felt very powerful – nothing could hurt me. But nothing could love me either. But I didn't care.

I don't exactly remember how the scene ended. I think I spent some time alone either in or on my cage. And when I came back downstairs and looked at my behind in the bathroom mirror, I was astonished to see two huge almost black circles. My butt was so swollen and hard. I got really unhappy with Master for inflicting so much damage. I figured I had a case of leatherbutt that would never heal.

But as the bruises faded – arnica gel works wonders for helping bruises heal more quickly – and I spent time thinking about the scene, I realized both my body and mind are a lot tougher than I'd thought. My butt was not damaged; it just took a little time to heal. And while the words we exchanged during the scene don't stick in my memory at all, I felt like I had vented out a ton of toxic feelings and it was over. Really, it wouldn't have been right for him to be angry at me for anything I said, because he worked so hard to bring it all out.

And then three years later, in typing what he wrote about it, I find out it was all a scene, not a punishment; that he was proud of me for standing up for myself; and that he was enjoying himself sexually – arrrgh!

I wonder how it will work next time – maybe I can just get mad at him for trying to trick me again, instead of him having to work up an excuse to "punish" me.

You know how hard it is to live with a sadist? His idea of fun is to set me up and then torture me for falling into his traps. Like the time he told me to follow him into the dungeon, and I walked right in behind him – breaking a couple of rules. So he punished the part that made the mistake, my feet, by hooking them up to his new TENS unit. It took me a while to realize he's not really mad at me for goof-ups like this (refer to his Masterism vs. Sadism essay in "The Lighter Side of SM" chapter), but that he's having fun.

And if I don't screw up, he'll make up a reason: "You folded my socks wrong. Bad slave. Get up to the dungeon."

What I learn in scenes with Master, he expects me to carry into everyday life. I've learned that pain won't kill me. It will hurt and feel unendurable, and there may be times when I more or less lose my mind for a brief period, but it will end. And after it ends, the memory of the pain will fade. I need to focus on what needs to be done to survive, and put the pain aside.

There have also been lessons in dealing with fear. I am learning to trust that Master always does have my best interests at heart, along with his own. I am learning to put my emotions aside and go along wherever Master wants to take me.

He gave me a very valuable lesson about two years after I had come to be with him. He knows I'm scared of heights. I think many people are, at some basic level – but for me, getting close to the edge of a building or a cliff always made me feel like there is more gravity and I am going to be pulled over the edge.

So, what does he do? Takes me skydiving. No warning, no clue until I saw the sign "Skydive Palatka." Five hours of classroom training later, we're up at 13,500 feet, and I'm standing in the doorway of a fairly small plane, two instructors hanging onto my leg straps, knowing it's totally up to me to say "Go."

I was looking down at the tiny, tiny ground so far away, and I was so afraid that I would die if I did this. And Master had said that it was my choice whether to jump or not. But thanks to all that Master had taught me about being rational when I need to be, I was able to put that fear aside and focus on what I had to do.

"Prop, up, down, arch!" and we were free falling. My focus was so close around me I couldn't see the ground or the horizon. I followed the procedures I'd learned in class and focused on keeping my body arched in the proper position for a free fall, and watching my altimeter spin (rather quickly) down to 6,000 feet. I think I had a little help actually locating my rip cord but I pulled it on my own at the appropriate time.

My instructors disappeared instantly, as they had continued their free fall to get out of my way and let me guide myself down. I remembered the next lesson, which was to stuff my rip cord into my suit so it wouldn't land on somebody or something below me. Then I looked up to check my canopy. Hmmm, the right side hasn't completely deployed. That's not good. Okay, reach up and try rocking the brakes like I was taught. Hey, that worked.

Now, where the heck am I supposed to land? Pulling one brake, I dropped into a spiral and finally located the drop zone right underneath my feet. I had almost five minutes of swirling around in the sky before it was finally time to think about landing. With the help of an instructor talking me down over the radio, I was able to brake hard and stall, coming in for a not-quite-perfect three point landing.

This experience was made possible only because of Master. He taught me enough about how to process fear and emotions and put them aside when necessary, and focus on what needs to be done. If it weren't for his earlier teachings both in and out of scenes, I wouldn't have had the presence of mind to clear my fouled chute without panicking.

And I have been able to work that backwards a bit, and take what I learned from skydiving back into other scenes – focus on what I need to do to get through the fear and let the rest go.

Later, he took me out for a celebratory dinner. I was feeling invincible, "If I can jump out of an airplane, I can do anything."

"Here, eat a frog's leg."

"Red!"

I thought it might be a good idea to go through a scene in detail, and share how I respond and try to process that pain Master likes to inflict, and how I see the way he controls the situation to keep my responses where he wants them.

Master was invited to give a presentation on pressure points at a club in Atlanta, 1763. This is a great place to go and scene, and we've been to several events there. Whippersnappers, the organization that invited him, was full of very nice and fun people. After his workshop, there was a dungeon party. We'd spent some time watching other scenes, and since we were both getting over rotten colds, I didn't think we'd be scening.

Master grabbed his floggers just to have something in his hands to play with while he watched other scenes. He hopped up on an unoccupied spanking bench and I sat on the floor in front of him. He started flogging the top of my head and dangling his floggers in my face. Then he said, "How about a nice flogging?" He'd offered me one of those before, with warmup and everything, and I'd really processed it well and enjoyed it.

He led me over to the huge slatted semi-circle on which he'd bitten the heck out of me at Spring in the South earlier that year – nothing like fond (and scary) memories to get the energy flowing. I climbed partly up the structure, bracing my body so my butt was well-presented for a flogging.

It was a relatively mild start (for Master) but as he intensified it, my top half would arch up, and he would put me back down. I tried to hold my position and used all the pain processing techniques I could think of. I focused on my mantra: *love brings pain pain brings blood blood brings love*. I focused on my breathing. I focused on just holding fricking still and telling myself it's only pain and pain fades. I've been flogged enough to know that I probably wouldn't have a mark on my butt from the sting of it. However, it still hurt a lot and it was impossible for me to stay still and keep my body relaxed for very long at all.

As the flogging intensified, I started to get scared because I wasn't processing as well as I "should have been." Arrrgh – why do I worry about what should be, instead of accepting what is? I remembered Master telling me once that I'm scared of pain – I'd first thought he meant pain physically, but I know how far from damage pain can be, so I'd disagreed with him. Later I realized the fear was about where pain takes me emotionally.

Impact upsets me. I get angry at myself for not being able to process it, then I get mad at Master for hitting me too hard to process. There are times I have hated him with all my heart for the pain he was inflicting on me. It doesn't last past the scene, but I still feel bad for hating or being angry at the Master I love.

So Master was flogging me harder and harder, and I'd keep arching up and he'd keep putting me down by touching my back with a flogger handle. Finally he told me to stay still. I tried.

I focused on my hand, just hanging it through the slats and keeping it relaxed. I tried to pour all of my awareness into my hand, just feeling the relaxation in my hand. I lost that battle fairly quickly and started to cry a bit from frustration.

He started the roller coaster ride, working me up intensely with the floggers, then doing something nice, like pressing his face into my nicely warmed butt. That wasn't exactly relaxing, as I was afraid he would bite me. He teased me about it though, and laughed as he felt my anxiety.

At one point as he ramped it up again, I curled my right leg up. He decided to correct me by pressing the pointy end of his flogger into my calf and holding it there. I could feel the intent to correct me and remind me to stay still. That's when I really started to bawl, not from the physical pain, although it hurt a lot, but because I took it as a punishment for failing Master. (I take it a lot more deeply than he means it, most of the time.)

He popped up to my head level and told me he hadn't done anything to make me cry. I disagreed, but that did me no good.

He flipped me over and started nipping at my nipples. In the state

I was in, I was so agitated, fearing pain when he wasn't biting all that hard. It was a waste of energy and I told myself to relax and stay rational. Then he broke into tickling me. I HATE being tickled. It's fricking annoying and it makes me laugh when I want to be serious, so that makes it even more annoying.

Master worked his way back down off me and the piece of equipment. He spread my legs wide, then he started flogging the insides of my thighs. He didn't go real hard at first, but that's a sensitive area for me, both physically and emotionally. I got mad and took it better for a little bit, then he ducked in and started nibbling – again it wasn't that hard, but I was remembering the previous scene on that same piece of equipment – Master was all teeth and I'd had to stuff my t-shirt in my mouth so as not to scream too much and disturb people. This time I had no t-shirt.

Master was taking me up and down and varying between pain I hated and intense sensations I liked and tickling and talking to me. I was a jumble of emotions and resented him for being able to so easily manipulate me. By bouncing all over the place, I couldn't find a focus to get me "out of there" mentally. Of course, that's not what he wants anyway. What fun is there for him when he's being a sadist if his bottom is not responsive?

So part of me is happy because he's feeding his beast. I'm still sometimes debating whether it's better for me when he scenes hard with someone else then brings the sexual energy back to me – or whether I really am happy to be both dinner and dessert. Though in this case, due to the rules of the club and the fact that we didn't have a private hotel room, I figured dessert would not be served that night. How does that man do it?

So he'd flog my inner thighs, sometimes using the point of one flogger to hold my leg open so he could have a better target, sometimes Florentine flogging both at the same time, popping in for a quick nip here and there and then popping up to mess with my head, asking why I'm flinching and crying. I told him I remembered our last scene on this, but didn't have a t-shirt to eat so he took his off and handed it to me. I noticed I was still enough in my own head to appreciate the view. A bit more flogging as I stifled my cries with his

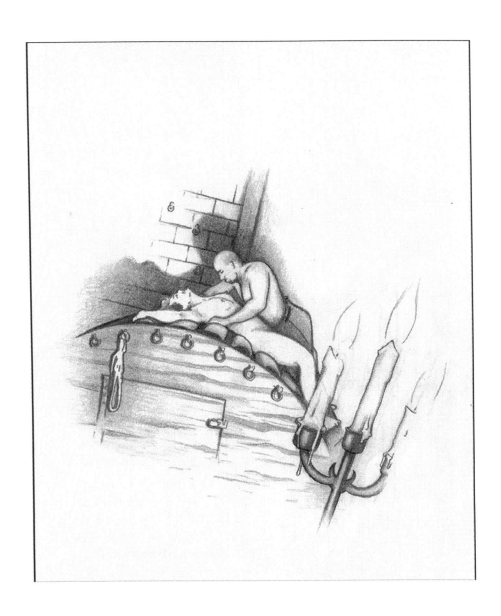

shirt, then he was back to reclaim it, claiming he was cold. Meanie.

The humor and conversation interspersed with what to me was a more than adequate amount of pain really kept me off balance, but it was fun for me at the same time.

I remember saying "no" a lot – I didn't want him biting my thighs or flogging my – ridiculous, hard to find the right word – after all this time in the Scene, I'm still shy – panties.

He usually ignores me when I say no. That's our dynamic, and it doesn't work for everyone. When I say no, I usually mean it with everything I've got. *No, I can't take it. No, it hurts too much. No, I don't want you to hurt me there.* I'm glad it doesn't matter because we'd never have any fun if he listened to me. Anyway, I'm not really saying no to Master, but to pain.

He popped up again and repositioned me so he was sitting on my thighs with my feet braced on a slat so he wouldn't slide off. He put his floggers down, one on each side of my arms, which were stretched over my head.

He grabbed my sides and started tickling again – my body convulsed and I knocked his floggers off to the sides. One would have gone over the edge if I hadn't caught it. Heart attack city for me – last time I'd caught a falling flogger I'd gotten beat pretty good with it. (Hey, maybe that wasn't a real punishment, either, but an excuse for Master to beat me – it worked well for me because I had something emotional to focus on – failing to follow instructions – which made the pain easier to take.)

This time, as I was cringing because of the last time (third time I flashed to another scene during this scene – reminding myself maybe it's best if I just stay in this scene), he just repositioned the floggers and went on with the tickling.

Later, with him sitting on me, having taken his glasses off, I told him, "I can still see you in there." I was referring to the way I used to not be able to see anything human in his eyes when he would be sadistic. I don't know if now I have enough trust and knowledge to see past the deadness he used to project, or if he just doesn't project it at me any longer.

He started punching me in the stomach, which upsets me, and

slapping me in the face, which makes me happy because it's sooooo wrong, and hitting me on top of the head, which for some stupid reason makes me laugh.

I tensed and did what I could to protect myself without actually resisting, but Master intensified it. Flashback number four to a Denver hotel room scene where he was hitting me in the stomach and I told him he was breaking my soul.

I sat up, careful not to dislodge Master from his perch on my legs, and he lightly headbutted me in the forehead to get me to lie back down. There went flashback number five, mean stepfather – but that lasted less than a second and I realized I was quite happy with Master for defusing yet another trigger – I really could have gone off emotionally about past abuse, but didn't, thanks to Master working so hard to teach me that the past is over and doesn't need to affect the present. I guess I spared us both some emotional fallout. That's not to say I don't on some level want to go "back there" and I'm sure we will some day, but today wasn't the day.

Master gave me his floggers to hold and as he'd punch me in the stomach and my body would contract, my hands would come up. With the floggers in them, I'm sure it looked threatening. He was teasing me about wanting to hit him and I remember trying to reassure him that I didn't want to – though I'm sure the handles came close to him a few times.

Yes, there have been times I have wanted to hit Master in a scene. Fortunately, I have either retained enough self-control or Master has restrained me. Restraints are important when pushing the agony state of pain because I do think there are times when I could lose control. Master hasn't pushed me that far, but he has pushed me enough to want to hurt him. Frankly, I am scared of the rages he has awakened in me at times.

Master flogged my nipples with the tips of the floggers and I mostly processed that okay, and some more nipping. Grrrr.

And more stomach punches, harder and awful.

Sometimes when the pain gets too intense, I turn to despair. *It's hopeless, I'll never be able to process it, never go anywhere.* It's really negative and I don't like to go there, but it is one way that I do somehow make it hurt less physically – by making it hurt more emotionally. Master has told me that this is a stage that some must pass through to get to something deeper, so I trust that I will come through the other side of it, but it is a very dark place to be.

In frustration, I said to Master, "I'm such a fucking weenie." He bent closer and made me repeat myself.

"You just swore at me. Are you allowed to swear?"

"No, Master."

"Then why did you swear at me?"

"I didn't swear at you, I swore at me."

"Nope, you swore at me, and you are not allowed to do that."

For once, I really wasn't upset at being reprimanded. My friend Neptune says sometimes you gotta' know when to break the rules. This was one of them.

It snapped me out of the self-pity and despair I'd been feeling, and got me reconnected at a more positive level with Master, and gave him an excuse to cause more pain.

He moved up my body a little and started to hit my solar plexus area. My body reacted instinctively – Master has taught me to realize that the body will protect itself when threatened, and the solar plex is one of those dangerous places. In my brief formal martial arts training, I was taught to aim for the solar plex to hurt and disable an opponent.

So Master, switching from a painful spot to a spot my body reacts to as a "danger" spot, took me from a "do your best to take it, it's only pain" headspace to almost a "fight or flight" mode. My mind may know he won't harm me, but my body doesn't. I curled up as much as I could and realized I was suddenly very nauseous. Now this was my body's genius defense mechanism – Master didn't feel like getting thrown up on then (though normally vomiting is not a safeword for him) so he slid off me and grabbed my ankles and pulled me down after him. A few burps and I was feeling better, but he decided it was enough.

He held me for a moment, kissed me and whispered, "I love you." Then he playfully slung his floggers over my shoulders, picked my shirt up and handed it to me with his toes and ran off to get cleaning supplies. I stood there, a little bit upset that he would clean the equipment – I'm the slave; that's my job.

Okay, I need to re-think that – Master was being sweet and letting me pull myself back together. He wanted to clean the equipment. Who am I as his slave to say he can't? Silly me. Thank you, Master.

So Master helped me get my clothes back on, wrapped me in my fuzzy blanket that my friend Dottie embroidered with Master's mon and my name, and I snuggled at his feet and glowed for a while.

A little later, as Master was wandering around the dungeon and I was relaxing leaning against the chair he'd been sitting in, I heard that question again: "So, if you're not a masochist, why do you let him do that to you?"

Maybe I can come up with a bit more of an answer.

While I don't *enjoy* pain, I do feel good after a heavy scene. For me, it's not about the pain, but about the intensity, connection, and passion that come with it.

Pain gives me a break from the mundane aspects of my life. During a heavy scene, my mind is focused on pain and pain alone. There is no room for worrying about the tasks that make up much of my day. Pain makes me focus and feel fully alive in the moment.

After the pain, and before the rest of the world starts up again, comes peace. I'm wrapped in Master's wings, safe and loved. He's relaxed, and usually snoring softly. I'm warm, glowing, and spent. Often I feel cleansed, relieved, and renewed. I feel strong. I feel spiritual. The deep connection Master and I share has been brought to the surface. I am content.

Peace is not something I feel very often. I'm wound pretty tight most of the time. I have a lot of responsibility – much of which I take on myself, rather than just doing what Master has asked of me. There's always something to be cleaned, checked, answered, or fed – but after a heavy scene there's a time when I can just be. As a service-oriented slave, I don't seem to be able to relax until Master is taken care of. I know it's not always what he asks of me; there are times when he wants me to take what I need without thinking of him, but I'm still not very good at that.

I didn't see clearly that pain brings peace for me until I read what

Master wrote about going to a place where he can just be – I realized then that I do have my own times when I too let go, and it takes pain for me to get there. Sometimes I carry that peace with me for a while, and sometimes I pull it up again later.

The more I think about it, the less I think I need to understand why, but just accept that I am what I am, and that being the slave of a sadist does make me happy. It's more than loving Master.

It's more than enduring pain to make him happy. I guess if there has to be a short answer, it's "because I feel so good when it stops."

After our last weekend in Atlanta, with the heavy scene I described above, we spent a couple days in the mountains rock climbing and camping. We were snuggled down in the back of his Jeep, and I was feeling a bit, um, pent-up. Neither of us had any release while we were at the event, so, having planned ahead, I pulled out a battery-powered vibrator. Master said, "Okay, I'll be nice," and allowed me to suck his cock while I masturbated. I, as usual, got distracted and spent more focus on him than myself. After he came, I snuggled in his arms and started concentrating on myself again, and it felt good but I wasn't exactly getting close to orgasming. After a little while, Master reached for my nipples and started tugging on them, fairly painfully. Within two minutes I had a very nice orgasm.

As Master rolled over to go to sleep, I heard the grin in his voice as he said, "Masochist."

The Aftermath

As I pondered what to call this chapter, terms like the traditional "Aftercare" came to mind. Then I thought about calling it "New Beginnings." But I settled on "The Aftermath" because of the images of people just after my scenes. There they lie on the floor, covered in sweat, tears, and snot, looking like they just went to hell and back. So yeah, aftermath is a good term, I think. What I will talk about is what goes through my head and heart after taking people into the abyss. Personally, I think the consensual sadist needs as much, if not more in some cases, aftercare than the bottom. This is simply because we are doing things to people that they don't like.

What I offer to my bottoms is aftercare for life, the term of my life that is. I have an open invitation to anyone I have ever done a scene with to contact me should issues or concerns ever arise. This is the least that I can offer the man or woman who lets me push them beyond their limits. Some of my follow-up is nothing more than a simple hug after the scene. Other aftercare has taken months of emails. Later, I will elaborate on specific situations that relate to a gamut of circumstances.

I have been asked to perform a variety of scenes designed to help people. You read about my reasons for doing the various "extreme scenes" that I have done. Often I only ask "why" of my partners as part of my own aftercare. So I guess my aftercare begins before my scenes ever do. Again, when I say *my* aftercare, I am talking about what I need to help me feel my partners are "happy" with what we are about to do or what we just finished.

It is not often that I say "no" to a scene. In order for me to do a scene, the reasons why a person wants to do it have to be similar to my own reasons. At one point I was asked to do a "Flesh Hooks and Suspension" class for an organization. A potential suspendee sent me an email stating their desire to be suspended. Amongst the reasons was "consensual sadomasochism." I don't do hook suspensions for sadistic reasons. Well, unless it is my slave, I mean. So I told this person that I would not do this if that were the reason. Again the aftercare began even before the scene. If we can't be comfortable with every aspect of a scene beforehand, we will never be comfortable with the aftermath.

But it can be hard to say "no" to someone. It is never my intent to hurt anyone in that way. But to fully address aftercare, we must address those issues and concerns that may prevent poor aftercare.

There have been two instances in my life when I was so totally put off by a person that there was no chance of ever doing a scene with them. Remember that I must love and care for a person to do a scene with them. So if you rub me the wrong way, forget it. This is true for all of us, I think. You can tell a lot from a person just by how they ask you to scene.

I was teaching at an event in Atlanta for the third year in a row. Over the years, I had made many friends there, one of whom was Art, a dear sweet gay male in his sixties. Now even though Art was in his sixties, he had the body of a thirty-year-old. I mean this man was in shape. And he had a most intriguing way of greeting me. As we would hug hello, he would ask, "Sir, may I pick you up?"

With my consent, he would grab my butt with both hands and pick me up completely off the ground – all two hundred pounds. Then he would bounce me up and down a couple times. I can assure you the first time he asked, I was a bit reluctant because I didn't know if "pick you up" was an invitation to take me home. Art and I have a great friendship and we scene each time I am in Atlanta to teach for his organization. Art is an awesome flogging bottom and can really take a beating. Each time we did a scene, I pushed him a bit further over the edge.

The last time we scened, after our session had ended and we sat leaning against a wall, Art was having uncontrolled jerking and shaking. He found it a bit nerve-wracking, I think. His legs would begin to shake and he would grab his knees in an attempt to make them stop.

"You know you can't control that," I said as I laughed at him.

"But it is really weird; I never had that before," he uttered, laughing also.

I placed one arm around him and my other on his knee as we laughed and enjoyed being together.

"I think you have a fan," Art whispered to me.

Looking up, I saw a boy standing about fifteen feet away from us jumping up and down on his tippy toes – hand over head – with the biggest grin on his face. The only thing missing was his shouting, "Me next, me next!"

I could not believe my eyes. Here I was in the midst of aftercare with my friend and I was being propositioned from across the dungeon for another scene. Yes, you get points for desire but no chance of a flogging due to your lack of respect for my friend and myself.

The next situation involved Hook whose story you have read. Hook came to Thunder in the Mountains the year after we performed his hook pull. I had never met his wife while I was in Hawaii. While walking around the dungeon on opening night, our paths crossed. Hook introduced me to his lovely wife and we began a conversation using our indoor dungeon voices.

Then along comes this young lady. Impolitely, she butts into our conversation to introduce herself, stating in her first sentence that she had attended one of my classes and then asking me for a scene in her second.

"Hi, it is nice to meet you. Um …. I am sort of talking to my friend."

"Oh, I'm sorry, I just wanted to let you know you can do things to me if you want to."

So do you think I "did things" to her? Nope. Again, I can understand and appreciate her willingness to bottom. But that is not how you go about asking.

I firmly believe that how one acts prior to a scene is a reflection of how they will be after a scene. Thus, I foresee how they will treat me after I have poured my heart and soul into them. For the most part, people know what they are getting into with me. If people take the time to know me, or anyone for that matter, they would know many do not respond well to these kinds of advances.

As I mentioned before, my aftercare begins before any scene does.

In the cases of the chapters written by my bottoms and my slave, most of them knew that they would be writing their thoughts at some point. More often than not, the writing takes place months after the interactions – it can take that long to get one's thoughts together, particularly if the event drastically changed the bottom's life. The writings allow me to see their side of it, both good and bad. Yes, the bad of it, too. That word still rings in my mind when I think about Rich.

The scene with Rich impacted me as much as it did him. You see, for the longest time I would not let people read about what happened to Rich's arm. Let me backtrack again. Following the scene with Rich, I did not scene heavily for a period of time, but when I did again, bottoms were required to read Rich's story. But what they read was not the version contained in this book. I took out the part about the severity of his injury.

Even as I write this, I examine my reasons for doing that. After all, it was an accident. Could it have been prevented? Maybe. For the longest time after that scene, I attempted to accept responsibility for his injury. But Rich would not let me. I offered to pay for his insurance out-of-pocket. Again Rich refused, stating it was not my fault. Clearly Rich had forgiven me for the accident. But I would not forgive myself. This was the first time anything adverse had happened in one of my scenes. Certainly, both Rich and I knew the risks involved, and the possibility of injury was and is always there. Just as there is danger in driving a car, danger exists in SM activities.

Even though I had taken out the part about how Rich got hurt, I told people about it. Maybe it just seemed easier for me to tell people about my actions instead of having them read Rich's words. Going into the scene, I think we both knew it would be a once-in-a-lifetime event. Rich and I have never done a scene together again. Neither of us have ever regretted our time together. But after a scene like that, there is really no place to go. That was one of the scenes where the top and bottom both needed mass amounts of aftercare; Rich's being largely physical and some emotional, mine being emotional and spiritual.

Part of the aftercare Rich gave me came in an email nine months after our scene. He wrote, "There is something I just realized and it is that if I had it to do all over again and I knew I would be injured if I did it the same way, I would not choose to remove myself from the scene … instead, I would simply ask that you tie me so that I could not pull with the tendons in my arms. Obviously I do not regret the scene or I would choose not to do it at all. I would do it again … just differently, and that is an example not of pulling away but of learning to do it better. That is the point I want you to understand. Don't quit playing like this … Just learn from past mistakes and do it better in the future. If I were younger, that is what I would do."

Reading the stories of my partners teaches me more about people and life. It reaffirms that they were happy with the choices they made. When I get that email that thanks me for a scene, it lets me know they did not regret the choice to jump off the cliff.

Only in the more life-oriented scenes that I do, do I ask people to write about them. For the most part, I don't "require" people to write. But always they let me know they are "okay" after the scene.

I have never been afraid that a person would turn on me after a scene. Part of that comes from the selection process: choosing people I get a good feeling from. But that was not always the case. Early on I was perhaps helping people before I was really able to provide enough aftercare for myself. This is where it will get a little strange. Depending on your beliefs, you may or may not understand or agree with this. For me, it was very real.

While attending an event in Orlando, I was approached by a young lady asking for a pressure point scene. We talked a bit about her likes and dislikes, medical history, and so on. I explained to her that what she was asking me to do would really open her up and expose her heart. She stated she understood and explained that's why she had sought me out. We did the scene, which involved crying and such, but was not about sex, rather an emotional encounter. After the scene ended, I felt very drained, even weak. The weakness progressed even further during the next few days. When I reported back to work three days after the scene, my co-workers acknowledged how pale I was. I had become physically sick.

About a week after the scene, the bottom sent me an email

thanking me and stating how much better she was feeling. She mentioned that her thinking had been clearer and her thoughts uncluttered since the scene. Additionally, she stated she had not smoked cigarettes or drunk alcohol since the scene. Apparently these were everyday activities for her. She claimed that her system had been cleared of all the bad that was in it. Well, if it was no longer in her, where was it? Many say it went into me, which they say is what made me sick. Later I was able to relate this story to Fakir Musafar, a modern Shaman, who agreed with the assessment that I had absorbed all the bad that came from her. Unfortunately, it took me some time before I learned not to take things into me.

The best way for me to illustrate this is to recommend you watch the movie "The Green Mile," starring Tom Hanks. What was astonishing to me was that these events happened to me long before the movie came out. However, in the movie there is a character who is a healer, able to extract illnesses and bad things from people. Very graphically, the healer coughs and chokes on the very thing he removes, then ultimately opens his mouth to let it pour from himself.

What I do now is spend time with myself after heavy scenes and the more life-changing journeys. I go for walks in the grass in my bare feet, climb mountains, or make stuff. These activities allow me to reflect on myself. They require my complete concentration. There is not room to think about the problems and issues of others. They also get me out close to nature and the open outdoors. As a side note, my slave sees an acupuncturist who opens the window of her treatment room to let out the bad stuff from people.

Comfort food is not really a phrase I have liked, but I must say there is truth in it, especially after a heated sexually sadistic scene. Perhaps I let out the most femme side of a female during her menstrual cycle, but I like chocolate after sex. This is a typical night in my home dungeon – scene till you are exhausted, which includes sex of course. Then fall asleep on the dungeon floor. Upon awakening, have chocolate ice cream. Other times, like at events, I load up on brownies and cookies after I am finished with a scene. Regardless, I have also learned to take in sugar and lots of fluid after scening, in addition to my alone time.

So enough about me. Now I will talk about the aftermath help I provide to my partners. As soon as a scene ends, my nurse mode kicks in. In a technical sense, when tops do any type of scene resulting in marks, it is trauma to the bottom. All SM people should have a degree of first aid knowledge. Being a nurse, I give bottoms very specific instructions on how to treat their wounds or marks. But not all bottoms follow instructions well. At times I have gotten emails a few weeks after a scene stating, "My marks are getting worse."

"Did you use ice, heat, and arnica gel, like I said?"

"No."

"Why not?"

"Because I like the marks, and I want to show them off."

Yes, we tops know you like the marks and some of you are only happy when you have some. But don't complain they are lasting too long and you want them gone because you have a family reunion to attend in a week. If you would have started to care for them when we told you, they would be gone before your family get-together. With certain implements that I have used, marks have lasted up to six weeks when they were not cared for properly. Please listen to the top when they tell you how to take care of your marks.

More overwhelming than applying ice to a bruise is mental aftercare. Most often is the question "Why?" *Why am I feeling like this? Why do I cry for no reason? Why do you make it hurt so much? Are you happy with how much I took?*

The question "Why?" stems from shattering limits and passing through the gate to the unknown. Because they walked the path to a new place, they have many questions, many of which only they have the answers to.

I find the major aftermath issue to be people looking for more answers outside themselves. The scene opened a new world of discovery, yet instead of continuing to look within themselves, they look to me for reasons why. It is then that I give no real answers, but offer understanding. You see, it is my belief that we all have the answers to our questions, our own questions, that is. I offer understanding to their questions "Why?" because having been there, I know what results. But I knew not to ask others "Why?" —

something I learned in martial arts. I offer them time to think about what took place, more time to look at themselves. They must find their own whys inside themselves, which is what the scene did – revealed them to themselves.

Another common question seems to be along the lines of "Was I good enough?" Let me just say there is a difference between a consensual slave, a submissive, and a bottom. In my opinion, Guy Baldwin explained it best in one of his classes that I attended, using the example of bootlicking:

A slave will lick your boots until you tell them to stop.

A submissive will lick your boots until they think they are done.

A bottom will say, "Lick your own boots after you beat me."

So when I talk about partners asking if it was good for me, it is the slave and submissive types. Bottoms tend to be the "beat me, fuck me, and leave" types. Service-oriented partners want to know that I got something out of the scene with them. Some worry that they did not take enough pain. For myself, it is not about how much pain a person takes nor how long the scene lasts. A sadist only needs to go to the level where the bottom no longer enjoys what is taking place. This can happen in a matter of minutes or as long as a few hours. I guess by default a safeword is when they are no longer enjoying it. But certainly one can be in an unhappy state before safewording. So in any scene where I am being a sadist and a bottom safewords, I am happy. Also if I end the scene, it is because I feel they have gone far enough and should not be pushed further; again I am happy. So have I ever been unhappy because I did not think a partner functioned well? Never. On the other hand, I have been unhappy with what a few partners have done with what they were given.

"Why do you make it hurt?"

"I am a sadist." Enough about that "Why?" question.

One of the most difficult aspects of aftermath has to do with coming back to the real world. There are many levels of consciousness most often referred to as subspace, that altered state of being induced by BDSM activity. I wish to elaborate on the returning from states to which Rich, Travis, and Hook entered. If you recall, what I told Travis when I brought him down from his suspension, "Now comes the hard part," you must understand they were all in a different world. While Travis interacted with a deity, Hook heard voices not of earthly presence. As I enter these states myself, states of peacefulness and painlessness, it is increasingly more difficult to return. It is a place where one wishes to remain – a state of feeling but not feeling, a place to just be. Perhaps if I have a fear, it is that my wish not to return will be granted one day. I dread the thought of being in a journey and not returning to my body. Is that what death is? I can't imagine what it would be like to witness death happen in a scene. To think what I put myself through because of Rich's arm. What would it be like for the facilitator to have me not return? Maybe that is why we do return.

But imagine being in a place where only love and no hurt exists. Then look at the world in which our bodies live. Each day you read of death and destruction. We face the uncertainties of jobs, money, relationships. Yes, the harsh realities of life can be difficult to return to; that is the hard part. How do we deal with life? I will not speak for others. Nor does what I think hold true for anyone but me.

Having made the journeys I have, I do think there is something else. What it is, I have no idea. But I have gone to another place. Part of my job is to help others learn of this place. I return so that I may help others obtain this peace. And if nothing more, my dream and hope is that we bring some of that peacefulness back with us to share.

My own aftermath care focuses on knowing that there is a purpose to this. I need not understand why, just understand that I can. There does not have to be the question of "Why can I do this and others not?" There does not have to be the question of why these things, these altered states, happen. Don't trouble yourselves with why, but ask yourself, "What can I do with what I have learned, and how can I share it?"

I told Travis it would be hard to return because he had never been where he was going. The first time tends to be hardest. And such events can happen without warning. You should prepare for this type of aftercare at any given time. This is easier said than done, my friends.

It is my hope that this has given you greater insight into the needs of a sadist after a scene. As you have read, you can go far beyond the need to know you are okay with them inflicting pain on a partner. There are many individual aspects to each scene. As such, aftermath care should be tailored to each encounter.

For my closing thoughts I want to say that "peace" can be found in every scene that involves suffering. This is to say every sadistic encounter I have, the bottom has the opportunity to grow, learn, and even travel in a spiritual world. But you must believe in yourself and let go of the physical world. Happy SMing.

~FifthAngel~

About the Authors

FifthAngel

FifthAngel has been involved in the rescue and medical fields as an ocean lifeguard, ski patroller, paramedic and nurse for over fifteen years.

His explorations into Sadomasochism (SM) began in the mid 1980's. Only recently did he become involved in public SM, in 2001. After his first public event in Orlando, Florida where Lolita Wolf purchased him in a scene auction as a top, he was recruited to present at TES30. Since that time he has become a sought-after presenter and educator for pansexual as well as gay leatherman organizations, events and contests where he is often asked to participate in "celebrity" auctions and fund raisers. He has presented seminars and workshops for numerous organizations and events throughout North America.

FifthAngel's traditional Japanese martial arts training began at a young age when he was groomed to compete nationally in fighting and forms competitions. He has been trained in the empty hand arts of Shotokan, Aiki-Do, and Okinawa Shorin-Ryu. His weapons training includes the bo, jo, sai, tunfa, nunchaku, and sword. In addition, he has received training in Shiatsu and the use of pressure points for self-defense. FifthAngel has obtained Dan rankings (black belts) in both empty hand and swordsmanship arts.

FifthAngel plans to continue writing and traveling to educate others about the many facets of his understanding and experiences with SM.

Contributing Author Rich Dockter

Rich Dockter is a leatherman from the Rocky Mountain city of Denver, Colorado and current director of Thunder in the Mountains. Rich came to the leather community about nine years ago after living a life as diverse as his sexual interests in the Scene. He graduated from law school in 1969, worked in the oil industry for many years as an oil and gas landman, owned a restaurant in which he served as a chef, and finally retired from a longtime position as national manager of credit and collections for a large magazine fulfillment corporation. During his earlier years, Rich married a woman and fathered a gay son. After an amicable divorce, he spent the next fifteen years in a primarily vanilla relationship with his first male lover, which ended with the death of his partner from AIDS and Hepatitis C in 1996. Rich himself is a long time survivor of AIDS and Hepatitis C and continues to fight that ongoing battle to this day. In 1997, Rich stepped into the leather limelight by running for and winning the title of Mr. Leather Colorado. Due to disagreements with the producer, he resigned that title and subsequently purchased the rights to Rocky Mountain Mr. Leather, the title under which he competed at International Mr. Leather.

Rich is also a member of San Francisco's Fifteen Association and the Chicago Hellfire Club, having attended both "Bootcamp" and "Inferno" during various years. He also counts himself as a member of UnCommon Ground, Denver's primary pansexual leather organization. He has presented many seminars and demos both locally and nationally for various leather events. Rich is considered a heavy player/switch in the Scene and involves himself in flogging, whipping, forced exercise, sounds, raunch, piercing, wax, and virtually everything else under the sun. In November 2003, Rich and his partner Brian Conway, traveled to Toronto, Canada, and got married. They live happily in Denver with their family, a Great Dane named Buffy and a Sharpei named Angel.

Contributing Author Travis Wilson

Travis Wilson has been an attorney since 1972, and in the Leather/BDSM lifestyle almost as long. He was Chairman of Houston PEP for eight years. He was a founder of the Houston S&M Ball, and was Chairman of the Ball for the first eight Balls, helping to make it an internationally known and respected Fetish event.

Travis has been a presenter at Leather/BDSM events for many years, presenting at such events as Black Rose, Beat Me in St. Louis, Tribal Fire, Texas Leather Pride, the GWNN Bash, Living in Leather, and many more. In April of 2004, he was the keynote speaker at the

Leather Leadership Conference Eight.

His writings about the BDSM/Leather Scene have gone "round the world", touching on topics as diverse as the intensity of the darkest S&M play, and the spirituality of hook suspension. He is also a jazz trumpet player who plays in both big bands and small jazz combos.

Those forced to listen to him may well consider that his most sadistic pleasure.

Contributing Author Hook

"Hook," a relative newbie to the BDSM Scene, has been exposed to some of the most prestigious events in the world like Thunder in the Mountains in his short-lived BDSM life. Although it is irrelevant to his contribution to this book how long he has been in the Scene, it is worth mentioning as it reflects that steps in personal growth and exploration have no bearing to longevity in BDSM. In fact the event he writes about took place at the first event he attended, less than six months after he first entered the Scene.

His interest in BDSM stemmed out of his 19-year marriage as a mutual curiosity between him and his wife. Growing up in Colorado for 25 years he now resides on the Big Island of Hawaii, a place that fosters personal healing and introspection. Living in the Hawaiian Islands for the last seven years, he has become a major contributor to the local Scene by promoting and producing national-level educators and events, as well as attending many local functions to broaden his own education.

For Hook, BDSM is the confluence of the spiritual, the sexual, and the profane, out of which a broader understanding of who he is flows.

Contributing Author and Illustrator Sherrye Segura

Sherrye has always carried herself as a strong, confident, dominant woman, for as long as she can remember. Some find her complex but she wouldn't have it any other way. She is a bisexual polyamorous switch, however she only gives occasional control to one person, Stephen, her primary partner of five years.

She also has a collared female submissive, Ayla, who has been with her for three years and of whom she is very proud. She is honestly thankful for each of her relationships and loves each one of her partners very much. They each give her something different and special that allows her to express and fulfill her needs and desires as a woman and in the BDSM lifestyle.

Sherrye (Lady BlackWidow) has been in the public BDSM community for almost five years now. She has been a staff member of The Crucible and Black Rose since her introduction into the lifestyle; and before moving to Maryland from Virginia, a member of R.O.P.E. She has been involved in the D.C. leather community behind the scenes for various events along the upper East Coast as either guest, volunteer, or staff including Black Rose, BESS, TES, Erotic Haven, Leather Retreat, Camp Crucible, Beat Me in St. Louis, Stars and R.O.B.E.

She has achieved a great deal of growth by being involved with the D.C. leather community and plans on being involved as long as she feels she can and has a need to satisfy her insatiable twisted desires. She believes that she has many more things to learn not only about herself but the BDSM arts as well and enjoys sharing her own play style and knowledge with others as well as giving back to the community as much as she can.

As far as past experiences, she has been a collared submissive/slave, dominant, and mentor and has explored both sides of the lifestyle. She has found that it has given her the ability to truly understand and relate to what a slave, submissive, and bottom experience and what it means to give and submit and exist in a power exchange relationship. She continues to explore in a realm all her own where she knows anything is possible if you can just imagine it.

Contributing Author slave leslie

In service to the SM community, she raises funds for the National Coalition for Sexual Freedom (www.ncsfreedom.org).

slave leslie describes herself as a pretty wimpy masochist, but very much appreciates bottoming to intense pressure point play and heavy piercing scenes. Full-body flesh hook suspensions and hook-and-chain bondage have developed into some of her favorite spiritual pursuits.

In other areas of BDSM, leslie enjoys roleplay as Snuffy, a very playful puppy, and has been exploring ageplay as a four-year-old. The arts and crafts she made for her Daddy are proudly displayed on the fridge. Please note that roleplay is just playing a role, and has NOTHING to do with real animals or children.

Regarding consensual slavery, while the path isn't always an easy one, the rewards of love and discipline make slave leslie feel very fulfilled. She welcomes communication with other slaves and submissives, enjoying opportunities to discuss the unique problems, challenges, and triumphs found in the Master/slave lifestyle.

Illustrator Devin Wilson

A native of Jacksonville, Florida, Devin Wilson's youth was spent illustrating flights of fancy. During his years at Douglas Anderson School for the Arts in Jacksonville, his artistic skills matured in classes of Art History, photography, painting, sculpture, and printmaking. After four years of student shows and two awards for scholastic achievement in art, Devin designed and built a stage setting for Douglas Anderson's 1989 holiday performance at the Jacksonville Times Union Center. Later, becoming a member of the Jacksonville Coalition for the Visual Arts, his work was shown consecutively for two years at the Jacksonville Landing, earning him reviews in both the Florida Times Union by Sharon Weightman and the Folio Weekly by Ted Weeks.

Outside of the J.C.V.A., he ventured into tattoo design, tattooing, and even murals. His painting series, the "Temple of Sleepwalkers" was gaining momentum along with paintings and drawings exploring a darker erotica. Some of these erotic images were made into a line of greeting cards, currently being sold in Orlando, Baltimore, Atlanta, and Texas. The self-expression evident through erotic art became instrumental in defining what Devin was to become, an artist and gay Leatherman.

Some of Devin's recent credits include a CD cover commissioned by Jacksonville singer/songwriter Jay Dean, for Dean's CD "More Than You Know," released in 2000. January of 2002 ended Devin's painting and sculpture exhibit called "Alpha-Omega" shown at Fuel in Jacksonville. More of Devin's three dimensional work, life-size circus animals, were featured in an installation at the renowned Cummer Art Museum. Devin is also the illustrator for FifthAngel's previous book, "The Finer Points of Pain and Pleasure."

Currently, Devin is traveling to several leather events throughout the year, displaying and selling his work with partner and artist Ray Castro.

Photographer Barbara Nitke

Barbara Nitke is a New York voyeur who has been photographing SM lovers for twelve years. She is best known for her compelling images of SM lovers, celebrating their deep bond and intense passion for one another, which were published in 2003 in the book, KISS OF FIRE: A ROMANTIC VIEW OF SADOMASOCHISM. Her second book, ILLUMINATA: AN EXPLORATION OF SEXUAL RELATIONSHIP AND DESIRE will be published in Fall 2007 by ReganBooks/HarperCollins. She has served as the official photographer of many east coast scene events, and presents slide shows and photo workshops for both scene and vanilla audiences. She is a member of TES and LSM, an instructor at the School of Visual Arts in New York, and an alumnus of the adult film industry.
Articles about her and her work have appeared in the New York Times, Harper's Magazine, The New York Observer, The Daily News, Village Voice, New York Press, Time Out, San Francisco Chronicle, The Boston Globe, and other publications.

She was a co-plaintiff with the National Coalition for Sexual Freedom in challenging John Ashcroft (later Alberto Gonzales), Attorney General of the United States of America, and the federal Communications Decency Act (CDA) which regulates obscenity on the Internet. The case was lost at the Supreme Court level in March, 2006. She is currently at work on the formation of a national anti-censorship think tank with John Wirenius, pro bono attorney for the lawsuit.

Glossary

Acupoints – Anatomical points located along the **meridians** where **Ki** can be regulated. Also referred to as **pressure points**. Depending on the reference used, there are from 365 up to more than 2000 acupoints. These points are most often stimulated by using needles, heat, pressure, or suction.

Aiki-Do – A defensive **martial art,** in which the opponent's force is used against them.

BDSM – Parsed as BD / DS / SM, an umbrella term for sexual activities involving Bondage and Discipline (archaic), **Dominance and Submission**, and **Sadism** and **Masochism**.

Bisexual – a person who has sexual preferences for multiple genders.

Bo – A long staff used as a weapon in the **martial arts.**

Boi – Generally, a lesbian who sexually identifies as a young man.

Boy – An adult in the BDSM community generally identifying as a submissive male, though being of male gender is not a requirement. The term "boy" in the BDSM community does **not** refer to a male child.

Bondage – Restraining another's freedom of movement during a **scene** to provide or obtain sexual pleasure, usually by use of ropes, chains, leather straps, wrapping material, etc.

Bottom – The one on the receiving end of **SM** activities, who experiences sensations inflicted by the **top.**

Caning – SM scene involving striking the **bottom** with a rod traditionally made of thin, flexible rattan. However, both flexible and rigid rods made of bamboo and other organic and synthetic materials are also used.

Catharsis – The practice of relieving stress and anxiety by bringing repressed emotions and fears to the conscious mind and purging them.

Consensual slave – In **BDSM**, one who considers oneself to be the property of another, or one who devotes oneself to serving or following the way of a Master.

Cupping – A Chinese medical technique in which a vacuum is created to bring blood to the surface of the skin. Most commonly performed with fire and glass globes or plastic cups and a hand pump. When cupping is focused on **meridians** and **acupoints,** toxins are removed from the skin, blood, muscles, and connective tissue as a means of healing medical disorders.

DM – See **Dungeon Monitor.**

Dominance and Submission – A form of **BDSM** that emphasizes control and obedience. The infliction of pain may not be present.

Dominant – In **BDSM**, one who exercises control over another.

DSM-IV – Diagnostic and Statistical Manual of Mental Disorders – Fourth Edition, published by the American Psychiatric Association, Washington D.C., 1994. The main diagnostic reference of Mental Health professionals in the United States of America.

Dungeon Monitor (DM) – a person in charge of overseeing safety during an event at which **scenes** are taking place.

Edge Scene – Extreme **SM scenes** that challenge physical and/or emotional limits.

Escrima Sticks – A **martial arts** weapon thought to have originated in the Philippines, consisting of thick sticks usually 24 to 28 inches in length made of bamboo or rattan. They can be used singly or in pairs for attacking and defending. In **SM**, they can be used for **caning**.

Femme – Exhibiting very feminine traits, sometimes stereotypical or exaggerated.

Fetish – Association of pleasure or sexual gratification with a specific material, object, body part, or physical characteristic, e.g., leather fetish, shoe fetish, breast fetish, fetish for muscular men.

Fundoshi – Japanese-style loincloth.

Hakama – Long divided skirt covering the legs and feet. Used in the arts of **Aiki-Do, Kendo, Iai-Do**, and other Japanese **martial arts**.

Heterosexual (Het) – A person with a sexual preference for the opposite gender.

Iai-Do – The Japanese **martial art** of drawing the sword from its scabbard.

Kata – A Japanese term meaning "form" or set, a set routine of movements performed as solo practice by a **martial artist**.

Katana – A Japanese sword used as a weapon by the Samurai, the ruling class in Feudal Japan, 40 or more inches in length and typically wielded with two hands.

Kendo – The **martial art** of Japanese fencing.

Ki – The Japanese term derived from the Chinese word Qi, which means vital energy or life force. The absence of Ki is death. Ki is the force or power that gives life.

Knife scenes – A type of **SM scene** using knives or other sharp-pointed or sharp-edged objects – more often to inspire fear and anxiety than to draw blood. Knife scenes often consist of gently dragging the point or edge of a blade along the skin's surface without breaking the skin.

Leatherbutt – A toughening of the flesh of the buttocks, both in texture and sensitivity, resulting from a prolonged spanking or beating.

Leatherman – A gay man involved in **BDSM**, whose interests often include leather **fetishism**.

Martial Art – A fighting discipline designed to promote skill in combat and self-defense either barehanded or armed with primitive weapons.

Masochist – Among **SM participants,** one who derives pleasure or sexual gratification primarily from receiving physical or emotional pain.

Masterism – Describes the theory of Mastering slaves as it pertains to BDSM. Masterism is a term coined by FifthAngel to use as a comparison to differentiate between what Masters do and what sadists do.

Meridians – The channels located throughout the human body that carry **Ki**. Depending on the reference used, there are from 12 to 20 meridians. **Yin** meridians flow upward, while the **Yang** meridians flow downward.

Mon – A Japanese symbol, much like a house crest.

Moxibustion – The process of applying heat either directly or indirectly to an **acupoint**, usually for therapeutic purposes. Most often, the **mugwort** plant is rolled into cones and burned for this technique.

Mugwort – an herb also known as common artemisia or moxa, often used for **moxibustion.**

Newbie – a person who is new to the **Scene.**

Nunchaku – A **martial arts** weapon in which a pair of hardwood sticks approximately one inch in diameter and twelve inches long are joined by a chain or cord and used as a weapon. Often used in pairs. Nunchaku are traditionally thought to be a farm tool used to beat grain, rice, or wheat.

Out-of-Body Experience – An experience in which a person perceives the world from a location outside their physical body.

Paraesthesia – a perversion of the sexual instinct.

Play – (a term I hate) See **scene.**

Popliteal Artery – A blood vessel located behind the knee that supplies blood to the lower leg.

Post-Traumatic Stress Disorder (PTSD) - A psychiatric disorder often caused by life-threatening or abusive experiences.

Power Exchange – See **Dominance and Submission.**

Pressure Point – See **Acupoint.**

Qi – See **Ki.**

Role Play – A form of sexual activity in which the partners assume identities or relationships different from their own to create an alternate reality, e.g. a couple might act as Daddy and little girl, Teacher and student who needs a good grade, or even escaped convict and the Warden's wife.

Sadist – Among SM participants, one who derives sexual gratification from inflicting physical or emotional pain. In BDSM, sadists inflict pain on consenting partners.

Sadomasochism (SM) – The combination of sadism and masochism, in particular the deriving of sexual gratification, from inflicting or receiving physical or emotional pain.

Safeword – Signals used to indicate that a partner in a scene has reached a physical or emotional limit.

Sai – A **martial arts** weapon sometimes referred to as the "short sword," the sai was originally thought to be used as a pitchfork or plowing tool for planting seeds. Measuring 15 to 21 inches long, it is made from iron.

Samurai – The ruling class in Feudal Japan who were skilled in a variety of martial arts disciplines, particularly the **katana** (sword).

Scene – 1) When lower-cased, the interaction of a **top** and **bottom** during **SM** activities. At times this is referred to as play (a term I hate), work, or working someone over. 2) When capitalized, is synonymous with the leather community, comprised of those consenting adults of all sexual orientations who participate in **BDSM**, **fetishism**, **role play**, **power exchange**, and/or **sadomasochism**.

Seiza – A position often used in **martial arts** where one is seated with the knees together and the feet tucked under the buttocks. This position kinks the **popliteal artery**, causing numbness and pain in the lower legs and feet after a short time.

Shiatsu – A Japanese term meaning "finger pressure:" the technique of applying pressure to **acupoints** to aid in the regulation of **Ki**. A form of therapeutic massage in which pressure is applied to those points of the body used in acupuncture. Also called acupressure.

Shinai – A practice sword made from split bamboo lashed together with leather. Most often used in the Japanese fencing art of Kendo. Can be used for fairly extreme **caning** in **SM scenes**.

Singletail – A whip consisting of a long, tapered, flexible single lash on a much shorter, rigid handle, e.g. bull whip, stock whip.

Slave – See **Consensual Slave**.

SM – See **Sadomasochism**.

Spiritual – Of, relating to, consisting of, or having the nature of the spirit; not tangible or material. Concerned with, or affecting the soul.

Straight – Regarding sexual orientation, refers to a **heterosexual** person.

Submissive – In **BDSM**, one who is subject to the control of another, the **dominant**.

Subspace – an altered state of being induced by BDSM activity.

Switch – An **SM participant** who is involved as both **top** and **bottom** on separate occasions or sometimes even within a single **scene**.

TENS Unit – A Transcutaneous Electrical Nerve Stimulation device, an electrical device designed to help relieve chronic pain and popular in **SM scenes** for the sensations it produces.

Top – One who inflicts sensations upon another in a **scene**.

Tunfa – A **martial arts** weapon developed from the handle of a millstone, consisting of a grip attached to a longer, perpendicular length of wood.

Vanilla – Sexually conventional people or activities that have nothing to do with **SM**.

Vetwrap – A lightweight, self-adhesive support bandage generally used by veterinarians.

Wakazashi – A Japanese short sword used as a weapon by the Samurai, the ruling class in Feudal Japan. The wakazashi is 24 or less inches in length, and is also used for seppuku (ritual suicide).

Yin – The passive, female cosmic principle in Chinese dualistic philosophy.

Yang – The active, male cosmic principle in Chinese dualistic philosophy.

Made in the USA
Columbia, SC
18 October 2020